Psychosocial Effects of Screening for Disease Prevention and Detection

Psychosocial Effects of Screening for Disease Prevention and Detection

Edited by
ROBERT T. CROYLE

New York   Oxford
OXFORD UNIVERSITY PRESS
1995

Oxford University Press

Oxford   New York   Toronto
Delhi   Bombay   Calcutta   Madras   Karachi
Kuala Lumpur   Singapore   Hong Kong   Tokyo
Nairobi   Dar es Salaam   Cape Town
Melbourne   Auckland   Madrid

and associated companies in
Berlin   Ibadan

Library of Congress Cataloging-in-Publication Data
Psychosocial effects of screening for
disease prevention and detection /
edited by Robert T. Croyle
p.   cm.
Includes bibliographical references and index.
ISBN 0-19-507556-0
1. Medical screening—Psychological aspects.
2. Medical screening—Social aspects.
3. Health risk communication—Psychological aspects.
4. Health risk communication—Social aspects.
I. Croyle, Robert T.
[DNLM: 1.Stress, Psychological.
2. Diagnosis.   3. Risk Factors.
4. Anxiety—etiology.   5. Knowledge, Attitudes, Practice.
WM172   P97454   1995   RA427.5.P79   1995
155.9'16—dc20   DNLM/DLC   for Library of Congress   94-22279

9 8 7 6 5 4 3 2 1
Printed in the United States of America
on acid-free paper

Contents

Contributors, vii

1. Introduction, 3
   Robert T. Croyle

I   What Do We Know about the Impact of Screening?

2. Psychological Impact of Genetic Testing, 11
   Robert T. Croyle and Caryn Lerman

3. Psychosocial Impact of Cholesterol Screening and Management, 39
   Karen Glanz and Mary Beth Gilboy

4. Psychosocial Impact of Cancer Screening, 65
   Caryn Lerman and Barbara K. Rimer

5. Changes in Psychological Distress and HIV Risk-Associated Behavior:
   Consequences of HIV Antibody Testing?, 82
   John B. Jemmott, III, Catherine A. Sanderson, and Suzanne M. Miller

6. The Psychosocial and Behavioral Impact of Health Risk Appraisals, 126
   Victor J. Strecher and Matthew W. Kreuter

7. Understanding the Impact of Risk Factor Test Results: Insights from a
   Basic Research Program, 144
   Peter H. Ditto and Robert T. Croyle

II   Where Do We Go from Here?

8. Toward an Understanding of the Psychological Consequences
   of Screening, 185
   Theresa M. Marteau

9. Screening for Disease Detection and Prevention: Some Comments and
   Future Perspectives, 200
   Torbjørn Moum

Index, 215

Contributors

ROBERT T. CROYLE
University of Utah

PETER H. DITTO
Kent State University

MARY BETH GILBOY
Temple University

KAREN GLANZ
Cancer Research Center of Hawaii

JOHN B. JEMMOTT, III
Princeton University

MATTHEW W. KREUTER
University of North Carolina

CARYN LERMAN
Lombardi Cancer Research Center

THERESA M. MARTEAU
United Medical and Dental Schools
of Guy's and St. Thomas's

SUZANNE M. MILLER
Temple University

TORBJØRN MOUM
University of Oslo

BARBARA K. RIMER
Duke Comprehensive Cancer Center

CATHERINE A. SANDERSON
Princeton University

VICTOR J. STRECHER
University of North Carolina

Psychosocial Effects of Screening for
Disease Prevention and Detection

1

Introduction

ROBERT T. CROYLE

Screening for disease markers and risk factors is an important component of public health efforts in many countries. Screening in both clinical and community contexts is promoted as a cost-effective means of identifying individuals who have an increased risk for disease or who manifest early signs of disease. Identification of at-risk individuals allows health services to be targeted to those who are most likely to benefit from early intervention.

The justification for screening programs, especially when implemented outside of the traditional clinical setting, often includes several implicit assumptions about human behavior. For example, proponents of many screening programs assume that individuals who are notified of their risk status will respond "rationally" by initiating or changing specific health-related behaviors. For a generation of health educators, the Health Belief Model (Becker, 1974) provided the theoretical justification for this risk notification strategy. Perceived susceptibility to disease was presumed to serve as a critical motivator of preventive health behavior. Individuals who were unaware of their risk status were expected to behave in a more healthful way once they were informed of their vulnerability.

Ironically, just when the fear-drive model of behavior began to be widely applied in health education, behavioral scientists were embroiled in a lengthy debate regarding its validity. During the 1960s, social psychologists conducted numerous experiments to test competing theoretical propositions concerning the impact of fear on persuasion and behavior change. As theories multiplied and the database became more complex, health educators came to rely more on their own practical experience and less on psychological theory and research. Program administrators couldn't wait for answers from the behavioral scientists, and the theorists and practitioners went their

3

different ways. Consequently, the initial development of major psychological theories such as the Theory of Reasoned Action (Fishbein & Ajzen, 1975), the Self-Regulation Model (Leventhal, Safer & Panagis, 1983), and the Transtheoretical Stages of Change Model (Prochaska & DiClemente, 1983) were largely ignored by the public health community. This meant that population screening programs were often developed without any notion of how risk notification was supposed to initiate necessary changes in attitudes, beliefs, and behavior.

As public health policymakers began to embrace screening as a disease prevention and control strategy, a handful of investigators reported evidence of adverse psychological consequences of risk notification. Some of the earliest evidence was provided by studies of children who had been misdiagnosed with heart problems by parents or health care professionals (Bergman & Stamm, 1967; Cayler, Lynn, & Stein, 1973). Similar problems were identified in studies of sickle cell screening participants. Although the distinction between "risk factor" and "disease" was clear to public health experts, parents of sickle cell carriers often interpreted carrier status as a sign of illness (Hampton, Anderson, Lavizzo, & Bergman, 1974).

The landmark event of the labeling debate was the 1978 publication of an article by Haynes, Sackett, Taylor, Gibson, and Johnson in the *New England Journal of Medicine*. The authors presented the most compelling evidence to date that risk factor labeling can significantly increase illness-related behavior. Among the steelworkers who were newly identified as hypertensive, illness-related absenteeism increased substantially from the year before the screening program to the year after. Had the authors reported findings based on traditional psychological measures, their findings might not have attracted so much attention. Instead, they presented objective behavioral evidence that also raised concerns about the potential *economic* impact of high blood pressure screening programs.

Subsequent follow-ups of the same study participants provided additional evidence of adverse labeling effects (Johnston et al., 1984; Mossey, 1981), as did evidence presented by other investigators at a McMaster University symposium on hypertension labeling (Sackett, 1981). As additional findings were reported from other hypertension screening programs, however, the picture became less clear. Some studies provided evidence of limited labeling effects (e.g., Charlson, Alderman, & Melcher, 1982), while most of the larger studies yielded no evidence of adverse effects, usually defined as either absenteeism or psychiatric morbidity (e.g., Mann, 1984). A review of the hypertension labeling studies published in 1988 concluded that labeling effects could usually be avoided by providing adequate counseling and follow-up to patients (Lefebvre, Hursey, & Carleton, 1988). But what exactly is "adequate" counseling and follow-up? Two of the largest studies that disconfirmed the labeling hypothesis were clinical trials that provided care and follow-up beyond the norm (Benfari, Eager, McIntyre, & Paul, 1981; Mann, 1984). Thus, the question of when and how hypertension labeling effects occur within typical population and clinical screening settings remains largely unanswered.

This volume is intended to provide a comprehensive review and evaluation of empirical research concerning the psychosocial impact of risk notification. This broad and diverse literature is widely scattered across many disciplines and disease domains. Consequently, a major goal of this effort was to bring the literatures together into one volume so that researchers and policymakers within the many subdisciplines could benefit from each other's work. The outcomes that the book focuses on reflect the focus of most of the research: psychological adjustment and risk reduction behavior. Other potential effects of labeling that are frequently discussed but rarely studied empirically (e.g., social stigmatization, loss of insurance, impact on family members) are accorded less emphasis.

The authors that have provided their perspectives on these issues are the leading investigators in the area of risk notification. Both American and European perspectives are represented, as are various disciplines, including psychology, health education, and sociology. The authors were selected not only for their expertise regarding labeling processes and theory, but also for their direct experience with large-scale screening and prevention programs.

The contributions are organized into two sections. In Section I, the authors review and evaluate the published research concerning psychosocial effects of screening. The first of these chapters (Chapter 2) concerns the newest and most rapidly growing area of screening—genetic testing. In Chapter 3, Glanz and Gilboy review findings on the impact of cholesterol screening programs. Lerman and Rimer (Chapter 4) then summarize the work on cancer screening, including mammography. Jemmott, Sanderson, and Miller describe findings from studies on HIV testing. The next chapter reviews the work on Health Risk Appraisal, a comprehensive risk assessment tool that relies on the large epidemiological database concerning risk factors. The last chapter (Chapter 7) in this section summarizes a research program that has attempted to study initial responses to risk factor test results in a highly controlled manner. This analogue approach aims to uncover the psychological processes underlying appraisal of and coping with risk information.

I am pleased that two outstanding health behavior experts have provided their personal perspectives on the research reviewed. Dr. Marteau looks across the various disease domains in Chapter 8 to identify themes and common processes in the psychology of risk factor screening. Dr. Moum provides a public health perspective, raising ethical and policy questions regarding the aims and benefits of screening programs.

I am much indebted to the authors for their cooperation and significant efforts. Pulling together the diverse studies in the various domains was no easy feat. The contributors have provided an important service to the public health and behavioral science communities. Disease prevention efforts will benefit greatly from their insight and perspective.

References

Becker, M. H. (1974). The health belief model and personal health behavior. *Health Education Monographs, 2,* 324–473.

Benfari, R. C., Eager, E., McIntyre, K., & Paul, O. (1981). Risk factor screening and intervention: A psychological/behavioral cost or a benefit? *Controlled Clinical Trials, 2,* 3–14.

Bergman, A. B., & Stamm, S. J. (1967). The morbidity of cardiac nondisease in schoolchildren. *New England Journal of Medicine, 276,* 1008–1013.

Cayler, G. G., Lynn, D. B., & Stein, E. M. (1973). Effect of cardiac "nondisease" on intellectual and perceptual motor development. *British Heart Journal, 35,* 543–547.

Charlson, M. E., Alderman, M., & Melcher, L. (1982). Absenteeism and labelling in hypertensive subjects: Prevention of an adverse impact in those at high risk. *American Journal of Medicine, 73,* 165–170.

Fishbein, M., & Ajzen, I. (1975). *Belief, attitude, intention and behavior: An introduction to theory and research.* Reading: Addison-Wesley.

Hampton, M. L., Anderson, J. A., Lavizzo, B. S., & Bergman, A. B. (1974). Sickle cell "nondisease": A potentially serious public health problem. *American Journal of Diseases in Children, 128,* 58–61.

Haynes, R. B., Sackett, D. L., Taylor, W., Gibson, E. S., & Johnson, A. L. (1978). Increased absenteeism from work after detection and labeling of hypertensive patients. *New England Journal of Medicine, 299,* 741–744.

Johnston, M. E., Gibson, E. S., Terry, C. W., Haynes, R. B., Taylor, D. W., Gafni, A., Sicurella, J. I., & Sackett, D. L. (1984). Effects of labelling on income, work, and social function among hypertensive employees. *Journal of Chronic Disease, 37,* 417–423.

Lefebvre, R. C., Hursey, K. G., Carleton, R. A. (1988). Labeling of participants in high blood pressure screening programs: Implications for blood cholesterol screenings. *Archives of Internal Medicine, 148,* 1993–1997.

Leventhal, H., Safer, M., & Panagnis, D. M. (1983). The impact of communications on the self-regulation of health beliefs, decisions and behavior. *Health Education Quarterly, 10,* 3–29.

Mann, A. (1984). Hypertension: Psychological aspects and diagnostic impact in a clinical trial. *Psychological Medicine,* Monograph Supplement No. 5.

Mossey, J. M. (1981). Psychosocial consequences of labeling in hypertension. *Clinical and Investigative Medicine, 4,* 201–207.

Prochaska, J. O., & DiClemente, C. C. (1983). Stages and processes of self-change in smoking: Toward an integrative model of change. *Journal of Consulting and Clinical Psychology, 5,* 390–395.

Sackett, D. L. (1981). The McMaster symposium on patient labeling in hypertension. *Clinical and Investigative Medicine, 4,* 161–226.

I

What Do We Know about the Impact of Screening?

2

Psychological Impact of Genetic Testing

ROBERT T. CROYLE
CARYN LERMAN

Our knowledge of hereditary disease has increased dramatically in the past two decades (see Table 2.1). In addition, advances in molecular biology have led to the identification of genes for disease susceptibility and DNA-based diagnostic tests for identifying carriers of deleterious genes. As a result, programs for genetic screening and counseling have become widespread. The provision of genetic information in medical practice has the potential to facilitate patients' informed decision making about reproduction and personal risk modification. As such, these advances have profound implications for reducing the incidence of genetic disorders and for reducing morbidity and mortality through early detection of disease in individuals at risk.

The rapid proliferation of genetic screening programs has generated a burgeoning literature on the impact of testing and counseling. Many of these studies have focused on the impact of genetic counseling on participants' knowledge and reproductive decisions (see Kessler, 1989 for a critical review). Although some of that work is referenced here, we focus on research concerning the impact of genetic screening and test results on psychological adjustment. First, we review briefly the literature concerning the utilization of genetic screening. This information provides an important context for understanding the attitudes and psychological experiences of those who decide to be tested. Then, we review studies that examined the impact of genetic screening and counseling programs, including those offering prenatal diagnosis, carrier testing for recessively inherited disorders, or predictive testing for late-onset dominantly inherited diseases. Following this review,

Table 2.1. Examples of Single-Gene Disorders

Disorder	Characteristics	Incidence
Cystic fibrosis	Autosomal recessive disorder affecting regulation of membrane transport of ions into endocrine cells	~1/2000 in some white populations, very rare in Asians; over 160 mutations identified
Duchenne muscular dystrophy	X-linked recessive disorder of the muscles	~1/300 to 1/3500 males
Familial hypercholesterolemia	Autosomal dominant defect of receptor for plasma low-density lipoprotein (LDL); increases risk of coronary artery disease	~1/500 heterozygotes
Fragile X syndrome	Common form of X-linked mental retardation	~1/500 males, 1/2000 to 1/3000 females
Huntington's disease	Autosomal dominant neurodegenerative disease of late onset	Variable, 4 to 8/100,000; much higher in some small, isolated populations
Phenylketonuria	Autosomal recessive disorder that can cause mental retardation if not prevented by dietary treatment	Variable, 1/5000 to 1/200,000; most common in Western Europeans
Sickle cell anemia	Hemoglobin disorder; first molecular disease to be identified	Common mutation in equatorial Africa; ~1/400 African Americans affected
Tay-Sachs disease	Autosomal recessive deficiency leading to early death	~1/3000 in Ashkenazi Jews
Thalassemia	Hemoglobin disorder	Most common single-gene disease; common in Mediterranean and southern Asia

Based on Thompson, McInnes, & Willard, 1991

we discuss the recent development of tests for genes that confer susceptibility to cancer and other multifactorial diseases. Finally, we discuss
the psychological themes that can be abstracted from the data and
suggest directions for future psychological research.

FACTORS INFLUENCING PARTICIPATION IN TESTING

Numerous studies have been published concerning the attitudes of
individuals toward genetic testing. These can be summarized by say-
ing that most members of both the general population and at-risk
groups express very favorable attitudes toward and interest in being

tested. The range of tests studied is impressive, as is the consistency of the reported findings. To cite just a few examples, a majority of respondents have expressed interest in neonatal screening for Duchenne muscular dystrophy (Smith, Williams, Sibert, & Harper, 1990), carrier screening for cystic fibrosis (Botkin & Alemagno, 1992), susceptibility testing for colon cancer (Croyle & Lerman, 1993), and presymptomatic testing for polycystic kidney disease (Sujansky et al., 1990).

But do the high rates of interest expressed in these surveys lead to similarly high rates of utilization? They clearly do not. The data concerning utilization of genetic screening and predictive testing (often referred to as "uptake") are less extensive than those concerning attitudes and interest. The studies published to date suggest that surveys of interest can grossly overestimate subsequent utilization.

Perhaps the clearest example of the discrepancy between genetic-testing attitudes and behavior comes from studies of individuals at risk for Huntington's disease (HD). Several descriptions of attitudes toward predictive testing for HD were published in a 1987 issue of the *American Journal of Medical Genetics*. The proportion of respondents who said they would take a predictive test if it were available ranged from 63% to 79%. Commonly stated reasons for taking a test were the desire to reduce uncertainty and the need to plan for the future. Expressed intentions to utilize prenatal genetic testing were generally lower (Kessler, Field, Worth, & Mosbarger, 1987; Markel, Young, & Penney, 1987; Mastromauro, Myers, & Berkman, 1987; Meissen & Berchek, 1987).

An early report of HD test utilization was authored by a group of investigators at the University of Manchester (Craufurd, Dodge, Kerzin-Storrar, & Harris, 1989). As stated by the authors, "All but 17 (15.5%, 11 females, 6 males) of the 110 individuals contacted through the register either declined (86 subjects) the invitation or withdrew (7 subjects) after counselling . . ." (p. 604). Other centers conducting HD testing have also reported less utilization than expected. The data generally indicate that when people are asked about their interest in a predictive test that is immediately available rather than potentially available, level of interest is substantially lower (Jacopini, D'Amico, Frontoli, & Vivona, 1992; Quaid, Brandt, Faden, & Folstein, 1989). Quaid and Morris (1993) mailed a questionnaire to 123 people who had not responded 1 year after an offer for free HD testing had been made. Respondents were asked to rate the importance of 17 reasons why a person might choose to forgo HD testing. Sixty-six (54%) members of the sample completed and returned the questionnaire. The reasons that were rated as most important by the group were "If my risk goes up, so does that of my children," "There is no effective cure for HD," and "I may lose my health insurance." The first of these reasons suggests that the desire to avoid threatening information is an important motive. The least important reason was "The testing procedure is too burdensome."

Nearly all of the published studies of genetic-testing intentions or utilization are purely descriptive. Most are not theoretically guided, nor do they utilize any behavioral science theory to interpret the findings. The few studies conducted within a theoretical context have typically employed the Health Belief Model (Becker, 1974). For example, a large study of a Tay-Sachs screening program compared participants and nonparticipants and found that participants were more likely to perceive themselves as likely carriers and less likely to believe that positive test results would affect them adversely (Becker, Kaback, Rosenstock, & Ruth, 1975). In one of several papers describing a prenatal screening program for hemoglobinopathies, Rowley, Loader, Sutera, and Walden (1991b) used the Health Belief Model to predict the test utilization of carriers' partners. In this case, the beliefs of pregnant women were used to predict the utilization of their partners. Model-related variables that predicted partner utilization included a greater perceived seriousness of the disease and a lesser perceived burden of intervention. The latter measure was a composite index that included attitudes toward testing itself as well as abortion. The most important determinant, however, appeared to be one of the simpler variables assessed: partners were more likely to be tested if they lived with the carrier.

The avenue through which individuals are offered testing can have a significant impact on utilization. This is illustrated by the findings from a large study conducted in Great Britain. Watson et al. (1991) studied utilization rates among groups that were offered carrier screening for cystic fibrosis. When the service was offered via a mailed invitation letter, uptake was very low (10%). Acceptance of screening opportunities was much higher, however, when offered at general practice (66%) or family planning (87%) clinics.

The link between testing-related attitudes and behavior appears to be stronger within the domain of prenatal testing. The explanation may lie both in the distinctive screening practices of obstetricians and in the decision-making context of pregnancy. Obstetricians are more likely to recommend genetic testing to their patients than are primary care physicians (Shapiro & Shapiro, 1989). Therefore, those patients with positive attitudes toward testing may be more likely to act in accordance with them because of physician endorsement. In addition, expectant parents do not have the option of postponing a decision regarding prenatal testing. Because abortion is one possible outcome of prenatal testing, parents who are willing to consider pregnancy termination may be especially motivated to have genetic testing conducted as early as possible. On the other hand, many parents who choose not to utilize prenatal testing may base their decision on a belief that abortion is unacceptable (Marteau, Johnston, Shaw, & Slack, 1989; Wertz, Janes, Rosenfield, & Erbe, 1992).

PSYCHOLOGICAL IMPACT OF SCREENING

Prenatal Screening

Prenatal diagnosis of genetic disorders by amniocentesis has become increasingly widespread. The indications for this procedure include maternal age greater than 35, family history of a genetic defect or inborn biochemical disorder, membership in a high-risk population, or a parent who is a known carrier of a genetic defect (Finley, Varner, Vinson, & Finley, 1977). In addition, amniocentesis is performed for women with abnormal levels of maternal serum alpha fetoprotein (MSAFP), which indicates increased risk for a chromosomal or neural tube defect.

Unlike presymptomatic or carrier testing, prenatal testing by amniocentesis carries a small risk to the fetus, as well as moderate discomfort to the mother when the amniotic fluid is withdrawn (Milunsky, 1975). Thus, psychological responses to amniocentesis may relate both to concerns about positive test results and to the stress-provoking effects of the procedure itself (Astbury & Walters, 1979). The potential of this procedure to generate anxiety is of particular concern, as emotional stress during pregnancy has been shown to be associated with an increased risk of prenatal complications (Reading, 1983).

The psychological impact of amniocentesis has received a great deal of attention. One of the earliest studies on the subject involved a retrospective assessment of women who visited a genetics laboratory for amniocentesis (Finley et al., 1977). Following completion of their pregnancies, 157 women responded to a mailed questionnaire measuring concerns about the procedure and reactions to the testing process (80% response rate). The major sources of concern reported by the women included whether the result would be abnormal (66%), risk of injury to the fetus (60%), having to decide whether to terminate the pregnancy (49%), pain (36%), and possible miscarriage (30%). Despite these concerns, however, 94% of respondents indicated that they would have the test again for a future pregnancy and 98% said they would recommend the test to others.

The potential reassurance value of amniocentesis was suggested by two early prospective studies. Astbury and Walters (1979) administered the State-Trait Anxiety Inventory (STAI) (Speilberger, Gorsuch, & Lushene, 1970) to 28 women who were at risk for having a child with spina bifida, Down syndrome, or anencephaly. Significant pre- to post-amniocentesis reductions in mean levels of both state and trait anxiety were observed. However, the observed scores were still within the range of those obtained in normative populations (i.e., mean = 35.1; SD = 9.2) Speilberger et al., 1970). In another study, Beeson and Golbus (1979) administered the STAI to 36 women at high risk due to either advanced age or having a previous child with a chromosomal trisomy (e.g., Down syndrome). Women were evaluated four times: prior to receipt of amniocentesis, 9 to 12 days after the procedure, 23 to 26 days after the procedure, and 1 week following receipt of results. Anxiety levels were found to peak prior to the procedure and again immediately before receipt of results. Women with a previous trisomy child had more marked elevations in anxiety than women at risk due to advanced age. In both groups, however, anxiety was reduced to levels within the average range following receipt of normal test results (see also Phipps & Zinn, 1986a).

Fava and colleagues (1982, 1983) evaluated the psychological reactions of 50 high-risk women referred for amniocentesis. These women were compared with a matched control group of healthy pregnant women who did not receive the procedure. The investigators administered the Symptom Questionnaire, a self-rating scale that measures anxiety, depression, somatic symptoms, and hostility. This measure was completed at three timepoints: before amniocentesis, immediately after amniocentesis, and following receipt of results. Prior to amniocentesis, women in the experimental group reported higher levels of hostility and less somatic well-being than those in the control group. However, these differences disappeared following the procedure. In addition, levels of anxiety and depression decreased significantly in both groups of women at each measurement point. The results of this study suggest that reductions in psychological distress observed among women receiving amniocentesis may reflect normal psychological changes that occur in the course of pregnancy, rather than being a direct effect of screening itself.

The above studies examined women who had knowledge of their risk of giving birth to a child with a genetic abnormality, for example, women over age 35. For these women who initiate their pregnancy with some degree of concern, amniocentesis may be reassuring or at least neutral because the vast majority will receive normal results. However, this may not be the case for women who are referred for amniocentesis after the discovery of abnormal MSAFP levels (most of which are false positives), because many of these women initiate their pregnancies without awareness of increased risk.

Marteau et al. (1988) addressed this question in a study of women with very low MSAFP results who were referred for amniocentesis. The sample included women who were aged 38 and older and who were referred for testing because of their increased risk for having a child with Down syndrome. These women were compared with those under age 38 who had not been aware of their risk prior to receiving the low MSAFP test results. Among women aged 38 and older, anxiety was elevated following receipt of their initial test results but decreased to normal levels 3 weeks later following receipt of the subsequent normal results. However, among younger women, anxiety levels increased substantially following the initial false-positive result and remained significantly elevated, even after receipt of the subsequent normal result. In fact, the average STAI score for the younger women following the false positive was 53.8 (SD = 2.8), which is significantly higher than the norm and within the range of patients with diagnosed anxiety disorders.

Robinson, Hibbard, and Laurence (1984) also observed extreme anxiety in women with abnormal MSAFP results. However, scores on the STAI returned to normal levels following receipt of normal results of follow-up amniocentesis (see also Tabor & Jonsson, 1987). They also found that anxiety levels were significantly lower among women who reported more satisfactory social and family support.

A similar pattern has been documented by Mennie et al. (1992), who published one of the first studies on the impact of prenatal screening for cystic fibrosis. They found that distress increased significantly when pregnant women were identified as carriers. In the sample of Mennie et al., when only one parent was identified as a carrier, the chance of having an affected child was 1/640. Women who tested positive and their partners were invited for genetic counseling. The partner was then tested. Most patients were informed that their partner was not a carrier, and their levels of distress (measured by a 12-item General Health Questionnaire) returned to baseline levels. All four of the couples in which the partner was identified as a carrier requested prenatal testing. Only one of these fetuses was affected, and the parents chose termination of pregnancy.

A study of Phipps and Zinn (1986b) suggests that women's responses to amniocentesis may be influenced by their personality or coping styles. They evaluated levels of anxiety and depression in a group of women undergoing amniocentesis and a group of matched controls, using the Profile of Mood States (McNair, Lorr, & Droppleman, 1971). This measure was administered prior to screening, immediately following screening, and after receipt of results. In addition, the Miller Behavioral Style Scale (Miller, 1980) was administered to assess whether women tended to cope by "monitoring" or information seeking or by "blunting" or information avoidance. Among women undergoing amniocentesis, there was a significant interaction effect indicating a difference between "monitors" and "blunters" in their patterns of anxiety and depression over time. Differences between monitors and blunters in anxiety and depression were greatest immediately following screening and least after receipt of results. Within the amniocentesis group, monitors had higher levels of anxiety and depression at all three timepoints. However, in the control group, monitors and blunters had almost identical levels of psychological distress. These findings suggest that women's responses to genetic screening are mediated by factors other than the procedure itself or concerns about receiving abnormal results.

Although attitudes have often been examined as potential determinants of genetic test utilization, one study examined the effect of screening participation on attitudes. Faden et al. (1987) compared the attitudes of two groups of pregnant women toward abortion. One group was recruited prior to the implementation of a MSAFP screening program. The second group was composed of women who participated in the program and received normal test results. The women were interviewed by telephone and asked about the conditions under which abortion would be justifiable. For example, the respondents were asked if abortion would be justified if there was a very good chance the child would be born seriously mentally retarded. The investigators reported that women who had participated in screening were more likely than controls to perceive their own use of abortion as justifiable in three of the four situations presented. When asked specifically about a fetus that had a confirmed neural tube defect, however, 80% of the women viewed abortion as justified, and this high rate was not affected by screening participation.

With one exception (Marteau et al., 1988), the above studies do not provide support for significant adverse psychological consequences of prenatal screening. However, all of these studies involved genetic disorders for which the fetus was at relatively low risk. Consequently, nearly all of the women who participated in these studies received increased risk information that was later modified by follow-up tests. This is in sharp contrast to dominantly inherited conditions in which the risk to the fetus is 50% if one of the parents is a known gene carrier and 25% if a grandparent is a gene carrier and the parents' status is unknown.

In the 1980s, prenatal diagnosis for HD, a dominantly inherited disorder, became available. There are two approaches to such screening: (1) exclusion prenatal testing, which involves testing the DNA of the fetus without determining the genetic status of the at-risk parent (who may not wish to know their own risk), or (2) definitive prenatal screening, which includes determination of the at-risk parent's HD status. In exclusion testing, the risk to the fetus can either be raised to the level of the at-risk parent (i.e., 50%) or lowered to less than 3%. However, the fetus can not be characterized definitively as a gene carrier in the absence of data about the parent's risk status. Thus, if an at-risk fetus is carried to term, the child would share his parent's 50% risk. However, this risk would increase to a very high level if the parent later developed symptoms of HD.

These complexities of prenatal testing for HD have raised concerns about the possible psychological impact of screening at-risk couples (Tyler & Morris, 1990; Spurdle, Kromberg, Rosendorff, & Jenkins, 1991). For example, in the case where a child is known to share the at-risk parent's risk, the couple's anxieties about the future are likely to be heightened. Alternatively, many couples may decide to terminate a pregnancy if the fetus is determined to have a 50% risk. The psychological sequelae of abortion of a fetus with uncertain risk are as yet unknown. Descriptive reports of couples referred for exclusion testing for HD have called for intensive counseling to educate couples about these issues and to minimize negative emotional reactions (Tyler, Quarrell, Lazarov, Meredith, & Harper, 1990; Spurdle et al., 1991). More prospective studies are needed to document the psychological consequences of prenatal testing for HD and other dominantly inherited conditions.

Carrier Testing

The purpose of genetic screening for recessive disorders is to facilitate informed decision making about reproduction. However, notification of an individual's carrier status also has the potential to produce negative changes in self-image and psychological status as well as social stigmatization (Massarik & Kaback, 1981). Despite this, few empirical studies have been carried out to examine the psychological and social impact of carrier testing programs. The importance of psychological reactions to carrier testing is underscored by reports that strong negative emotions can interfere with cognitive processing of genetic information and subsequent decision making (Antley, 1979).

The first reports of the impact of carrier testing were produced from a study conducted in a small farming village in Greece (Stamatoyanno-poulus, 1974). In this community, 23% of the population were carriers of the sickle cell (SC) gene and 1 in 100 infants were born with SC disease. A genetic screening program was initiated to screen the population and to counsel carriers about the disease. In addition, as marriages in this community were arranged, counseling was intended to facilitate discussion of carrier status in an effort to avoid matings between two carriers. A 7-year follow-up evaluation of the community indicated that notification of carrier status resulted in anxiety, embarrassment, and an inferior social status, particularly among women. In fact, 20% of parents reported that they requested that their noncarrier children not marry a carrier, even though this union would not yield any offspring with the disease.

To evaluate stigmatization associated with SC carrier identification, Wooldridge and Murray (1988) developed the Health Orientation Scale (HOS). This semantic differential scale assesses negative changes in self-image associated with carrier status and negative attitudes toward carriers in hypothetical situations. This instrument was administered to 199 participants in genetic counseling for SC disease; 136 of these were carriers and 63 were noncarriers, primarily relatives. No differences were found between carriers and noncarriers in the adjectives they used to describe themselves, suggesting that carriers did not have a diminished self-image. However, noncarriers were found to have more negative attitudes about sickle cell trait than carriers, suggesting that carrier status may be socially stigmatizing.

Issues of self-image and stigmatization of carrier status also have been examined with respect to screening for Tay-Sachs disease (TSD). For example, Childs, Gordis, Kaback, and Kazazian (1976) conducted a descriptive retrospective assessment of 346 couples who participated in TSD carrier screening: 128 carrier/noncarrier couples; 109 noncarrier/noncarrier couples; 52 couples with inconclusive test results; and 57 men whose pregnant wives were not tested. One half of carriers reported that they were upset when they first were notified of their status. In couples in which the wife was the carrier, she was more likely to be upset than her spouse. However, when the husband was the carrier, both partners tended to be equally upset. Despite these short-term reactions, the vast majority of carriers and noncarriers ultimately were relieved by the testing experience, and reported that it increased their perceived control over reproductive decisions.

Also, the vast majority of respondents reported that they discussed their carrier status freely with friends and family and did not feel stigmatized.

In a later study, Massarik & Kaback (1981) conducted structured in-person interviews with 74 carriers of the TSD gene who had participated in a mass screening program. Thirty percent of respondents reported that they were quite concerned and 21% said they were deeply troubled when they first were notified of their test results. Spouses of carriers tended to view the test results as less serious; 20% were quite concerned and 7% were deeply troubled. One year after screening, none of the carriers reported that they were deeply troubled and only 15% were still concerned. The investigators concluded that although TSD carrier notification may create some discomfort, there is no evidence of severe negative psychological sequelae or stigmatization.

Some of the effects of carrier notification may be too subtle to be captured by traditional psychiatric assessment instruments. Even when individuals do not report distress or other symptoms, specific self-perceptions may be affected. This kind of effect is illustrated by another study of TSD carriers (Marteau, van Duijn, & Ellis, 1992). Although the study found no differences between carriers and noncarriers in their perceptions of current health, carriers were found to have less optimistic views about their future health. This finding suggests that investigators need to broaden dependent measures to include a more diverse assessment of self-related beliefs and attitudes.

Recently, pilot studies of carrier screening programs for cystic fibrosis (CF) have yielded data concerning psychosocial effects. Unlike earlier screening programs that targeted high-risk populations, carrier screening for CF is being offered in Great Britain to the general population. Watson et al. (1992) reported a prospective comparison of carriers and noncarriers using measures of anxiety, reproductive attitudes, and CF-related knowledge. Carriers reported a small but significant increase in anxiety following testing, as measured by the STAI. Nevertheless, most carriers were not concerned about their result 6 months after testing. Long-term anxiety was related to fertility intentions. Almost all of those who did report some anxiety at the 6-month follow-up also reported intentions to have children.

The above studies have examined the impact of carrier notification on persons who were self-selected for participation in genetic screening programs. In a series of studies, Rowley, Fisher, and Lipkin (1979; 1984) evaluated the impact of genetic screening and counseling in a population where no specific informed consent for testing was obtained. This population included adult members of a Health Maintenance Organization (HMO) who were screened for beta-thalassemia (BT) trait as part of their primary health care. Carriers of the BT gene are at risk for having offspring with Cooley anemia. In an initial evaluation of this program (Rowley et al., 1979), 40 persons who had tested positive and 40 noncarrier controls were evaluated with respect to their knowledge, self-concept, and mood. Persons who had tested positive were randomized to receive either "conventional counseling" by a physician or "programmed counseling" involving a videotape of an actual counseling session. The results of testing and the implications of being a carrier were addressed during these sessions. Control subjects viewed a film on general health maintenance. Relative to controls, persons with BT trait showed significant immediate pre- to postcounseling changes in knowledge about BT and genetics, but no changes in mood. The effects of the two counseling approaches did not differ significantly, indicating that educational videos may be a cost-effective mechanism to provide genetic counseling in the primary care setting (Fisher, Rowley, & Lipkin, 1981). Finally, a follow-up study of 265 persons positive for BT trait demonstrated that the knowledge gains observed immediately after counseling were maintained at 2 and 10 months and there were no adverse changes in mood. In addition, a patient-oriented counseling approach was not found to have a greater positive impact on knowledge or mood, compared with the programmed or conventional counseling methods (Rowley et al., 1984). This lack of difference was partly due to a ceiling effect in that overall levels of knowledge and positive mood among those counseled was very high. This series of studies suggests that genetic screening and counseling in an unselected HMO population can result in improvements in knowledge without any adverse psychological consequences.

Predictive Testing

The availability of predictive testing for adult-onset diseases raises new psychosocial concerns and challenges. In contrast to prenatal or carrier testing to determine the risk to one's offspring, predictive testing is employed to determine one's personal risk for developing a disease later in life. In the case of Huntington's disease, an asymptomatic at-risk person may learn that he has a 99% chance of developing this devastating disease sometime in the future. The absence of options for risk modification or treatment for HD increases the potential for severe adverse psychological reactions to a positive test result. Linkage analysis, the method initially used for predictive testing for HD, poses other problems. It may be necessary to obtain DNA samples from both unaffected and affected family members—some of whom may not wish to know their risk or even to participate in testing. These circumstances may generate additional emotional stress.

Following the initiation of pilot testing programs for HD, several investigators sought to examine the anticipated reactions of at-risk persons to a positive predictive test result. Potential respondents, those at 50% risk for HD, were identified through local HD organizations and/or through mass media. Different modes of assessment were used in these studies, including mailed questionnaires (Mastromauro et al., 1987), telephone surveys (Meissen and Berchek, 1987), and semi-structured interviews (Kessler et al., 1987). In the study by Mastromauro and colleagues (1987), 29% of respondents anticipated that they would have suicidal thoughts if they tested positive for the HD gene, whereas 11% of participants in Kessler's (1987) study said that they actually would consider suicide under these circumstances. The potential for suicidal behavior among persons who test positive for HD is a valid concern, given that suicide rates in persons with diagnosed HD are 4 times higher than in the general population (Farrer, 1986). These concerns are not limited to at-risk persons, however. Partners of HD patients have been shown to suffer difficulties coping with the threat of HD to their children, as well as the mental and personality changes that can accompany the disease process in the affected spouse (Evers-Kiebooms, Swerts, & Van den Berghe, 1990). A recent study confirmed that suicide risk is elevated not only among individuals diagnosed with HD but also among spouses and other family members (Di Maio, et al., 1993).

A pilot predictive testing project for HD was initiated in 1986 in British Columbia. This program was designed to determine the demand for predictive testing and to develop interventions to manage the negative psychological sequelae of participation (Fox, Bloch, Fahy, & Hayden, 1989). Potentially eligible subjects, those at 25% or 50% risk for HD, are recruited through local HD societies and registries. The protocol includes a precounseling assessment of knowledge and attitudes toward testing, as well as a battery of validated psychological measures of depression, overall mental health, life satisfaction, and social support. In addition, all potential participants receive extensive education about the implications of predictive testing, rehearsal of strategies to manage potentially negative emotional reactions to a positive result, and a physical examination. Psychological assessments are repeated immediately following disclosure of test results and at multiple timepoints over the subsequent 2 years.

The investigators reported on the psychological characteristics of the first 51 candidates who registered for predictive testing (Bloch, Fahy, Fox, & Hayden, 1989). Mean scores on measures of mental health were found to be comparable to those of the general population, and overall levels of social support and life satisfaction were high. About 21% of candidates were at least mildly depressed, but only one person was severely depressed. Additionally, 33% of subjects indicated that they would consider suicide if they had a positive test result. However, none of these persons reported that they would be likely to take this action at present or in the early stages of the disease. The investigators concluded that persons who register for testing are not psychologically different from the general population and that self-selection for testing may result in a sample with better overall adjustment than that found among most persons at risk for HD. It should be noted, however, that one participant who was found to have early clinical signs of HD had a severe suicidal reaction, which required psychiatric hospitalization (Lam et al., 1988). Although this case is only one out of the 60 persons enrolled in the program, it underscores the need for sufficient psychosocial resources to manage the reactions of participants in predictive testing programs.

A major prospective study of the impact of predictive testing in British Columbia was recently published (Wiggins et al., 1992). All 135 of the study participants were at 50% risk of having inherited the gene for HD. They were administered a battery of psychological measures before, 7 to 10 days after, 6 months after, and 12 months after testing. The investigators compared those who were told they were likely to have the gene (referred to as the increased risk group) and those told they probably did not have the gene (referred to as the decreased risk group).

At the first follow-up (7 to 10 days after testing), scores on the Beck Depression Inventory (BDI), General Well-Being Schedule, and the General Symptom Index of the SCL-90 were all significantly different, with the increased risk group manifesting higher distress. These differences were due both to increased distress in the increased risk group and to decreased distress in the decreased risk group. However, these differences decreased at the 6-month follow-up so that only well-being scores remained significantly different. At 12 months, the two groups did not differ significantly. Additional analyses revealed significant declines in distress for both groups over the 12-month period.

An interesting feature of the Wiggins et al. study was the inclusion of 40 participants who did not receive information altering their prior risk status. Some of these persons did not want to take the test (23), whereas others were told that their test results were uninformative (17). Psychologically, these individuals did not fare as well as the others over the course of the study. They did not manifest the slight improvements in adjustment that characterized the other study subjects. At the 12-month follow-up, these subjects had significantly higher scores on the BDI and lower scores on the General Well-Being Scale than the other participants. At baseline, the three study groups were not significantly different on these measures.

Tibben and his colleagues (Tibben, Duivenvoorden, et al., 1993; Tibben, Frets, et al., 1993) reported data from a 6-month follow-up of participants in the Dutch HD testing program. The sample included 29 carriers and 44 noncarriers. A wide variety of measures were used, including the Impact of Events Scale, the Beck Hopelessness Scale, the General Health Questionnaire, and the brief version of the Social Support Questionnaire. The study yielded a number of interesting findings, only some of which can be summarized here. HD carriers reported more intrusive thoughts and feelings than noncarriers, but there was no difference on the measure of hopelessness. In many cases, the pretest measures proved to be significant predictors of posttest measures, whereas the effects of test result were not significant. The investigators attributed much of the self-report data from carriers to denial or minimization. One of the most important implications of their findings is that individual difference variables are more important in the genetic testing context than previously expected. The research also suggests strategies by which individuals who are at risk for adverse psychological consequences of testing might be identified prior to testing.

The British Columbia group has described in detail the experiences and psychological reactions of several individuals tested for HD (Bloch et al., 1992; Huggins et al., 1992). These case studies "were chosen to illustrate recurrent and common themes which have emerged during counseling and to highlight the strategies for coping with this information" (Bloch et al., 1992, p. 499). The authors interpret their case evidence as suggesting that psychological preparation for possible test results is an important determinant of psychological reactions. Seeking social support was a common coping strategy among those studied. One of the unexpected findings was the adverse impact of good news among some of those who were told they were unlikely to develop HD. For these individuals, who had lived their lives under the cloud of heightened risk, the prospect of a long life without the disease was both unexpected and unplanned for.

One of the cases described by Huggins et al. (1992, p. 513) highlights the role of individual perceptions as a mediator of psychosocial effects of test results. Like most of those tested, this 30-year-old woman had a parent with HD, which put her at 50% risk. As described by the investigators,

> She saw her 50% risk as an uncertainty that could go either way. She faced the dilemma of whether or when to have predictive testing. When she was told she has a risk of 11%, she said now *for sure* I have an 11% risk for having Huntington disease. It seemed like a certain fact, in contrast to a 50% risk which she interpreted as more uncertainty.

Huggins et al. reported that approximately 10% of those who received a test result that indicated a *decreased* risk for HD have needed additional counseling to help them cope with their new risk status.

GENETIC TESTING FOR CANCER SUSCEPTIBILITY

In recent years, a number of genes that predispose to dominantly inherited cancer syndromes have been identified. These include the genes for retinoblastoma, adenomatous polyposis coli, neurofibromatosis, Wilms' tumor, and the Li-Fraumeni syndrome, which is characterized by familial clustering of sarcomas, leukemias, brain tumors, breast tumors, and other malignancies (Friend et al., 1986; Vogelstein et al., 1988; Weinberg, 1991). However, such dominantly inherited cancer syndromes are rare. The majority of cancer cases are attributable to the effects of multiple genes in conjunction with environmental cofactors. For example, recent studies have identified lung cancer susceptibility genes that code for enzymes that metabolize chemical carcinogens including tobacco (Amos, Caporaso, & Weston, 1992). Other work has focused on genes important in metabolizing occupational carcinogens that affect the bladder (Vineis et al., 1990) and dietary components implicated in ovarian cancer (Cramer et al., 1989).

The mapping of some of these genes has made it possible to use genetic screening to identify persons at high risk for developing cancer. Although genetic counseling for cancer is becoming more widespread, there have not yet been any empirical studies to document the psychological impact of participation in these programs. However, numerous questions and concerns about genetic screening for cancer have been raised (Lerman & Croyle, 1994; Lerman, Rimer, & Engstrom 1991; Li et al., 1992). For example, the probability that an individual with a dominantly inherited mutation in a cancer susceptibility gene will develop cancer by age 70 ranges from 50% to 90%. Thus, identified gene carriers must live with significant uncertainty about their futures. Additionally, many carriers of cancer genes will be faced with difficult decisions about options for disease prevention and surveillance. Medical recommendations might include lifestyle changes such as dietary modification and smoking cessation, changes in patterns of surveillance including more invasive screening tests, avoidance of occupational exposures, and in some cases, prophylactic surgery. The psychological impact of communicating genetic information about cancer susceptibility must be examined, as negative psychological sequelae could interfere with adherence to recommended cancer prevention and control regimens. Information gained from this line of research will be applicable to other multifactorial diseases, such as heart disease and diabetes, where there are options for personal risk modification.

DISCUSSION

Research concerning the psychosocial impact of screening for genetic defects has provided a large and diverse collection of findings. In the discussion that follows, we attempt to integrate these data by describing common psychological themes that arise in the genetic screening context. We then identify some important gaps in the research literature. Finally, we discuss briefly some of the clinical and public health implications of these findings and the many questions that remain to be answered.

Psychological Themes

The importance of psychological preparation for genetic testing has been discussed frequently, but now it can be said that the empirical justification for this assumption is growing. The evidence suggests that risk information produces greater distress among individuals who were previously unaware of their risk status (e.g., Marteau et al., 1988). As genetic screening is integrated into routine clinical practice, it is likely that more tests will be conducted without prior informed consent. This is illustrated by the Rowley hemoglobinopathy project in Rochester (Rowley, Fisher, & Lipkin, 1979), in which most physicians authorized testing without consulting their patients. It should be noted that prior risk awareness has been identified in other screening contexts as a significant moderator of emotional and behavioral reactions to risk notification (e.g., Haynes, Sackett, Taylor, Gibson, & Johnson,

1978). However, previous research suggests that the benefits of preparatory information about genetic testing may depend on individual
coping styles.

A second psychological theme that is apparent is the desire to reduce
uncertainty (Decruyenaere, Evers-Kiebooms, & Van den Berghe, 1993).
Uncertainty reduction is often cited by screening participants as a
reason for undergoing genetic testing (e.g., Tibben et al., 1993). Thus,
it only makes sense that these patients are likely to be upset if test
results do not provide the level of certainty that they hoped to achieve.
This may be a particular problem when screening for multifactorial
diseases. The penetrance of such genes tends to be lower, since expres-
sion of the disease phenotype is influenced by environmental cofactors.
This issue can arise in many screening domains (see Lerman & Rimer,
Chapter 4), but it appears that individuals are especially vulnerable
to the myth that clinical genetic information is necessarily accurate
and predictive. This highlights another critical function of preparatory
genetic counseling: educating screening participants about the nature
and reliability of particular genetic tests.

Not only do patients want to reduce uncertainty, they also hope to
receive good news. This introduces a third psychological theme, goal
conflict. Many people want definitive and complete information, and
at the same time they prefer good news to bad news. Consequently,
emotional responses to risk information may be influenced by either
one or both of these goals being unmet (see also Ditto & Croyle,
Chapter 7). This is illustrated by Wexler's (1991) description of an
individual who participated in HD testing:

> Do people really want to know the truth? A woman came to our testing
> clinic, highly functional, intelligent, a working wife and mother, and la-
> mented that her family was not genetically informative enough for her to
> be tested. She stated that she would definitely like to be tested as this
> would help her advise her family better. This woman had been symptomatic
> for about five years but never diagnosed. Her statements about why she
> wanted the test were cogent and persuasive. She wanted to know the truth.
> Yet something in her very powerfully did not want to know the facts. The
> truth was that she functioned better in denial; when the denial was finally
> cracked by a clinical diagnosis, she and her family were devastated. (p. 87)

Goal conflict is especially apparent in the domain of prenatal testing,
where the desire to give birth only to a healthy baby can conflict
with the belief that abortion is immoral. Perhaps the most important
potential conflict, however, is that between the sponsors of a screening
program and its participants. For policymakers who take a public

health perspective, the primary goal of a screening program may be to achieve long-term reductions in disease prevalance through the prevention or termination of defective fetuses. In contrast, many parents perceive participation in screening as a way to obtain information partly for its own sake; some simply wish to prepare themselves about the pending birth of a child with special needs.

One of the important questions that arises when one examines the research on genetic screening is whether it raises psychological issues that are unique. When screening programs as a whole are considered, what is really different about genetic screening? Interestingly, this issue was rarely addressed in the literature we reviewed. Most of the articles on genetic screening are published in genetics journals and written for an audience of medical geneticists and genetic counselors. As a result, findings are not discussed within a broader context, and the literature on screening in other domains is rarely cited.

One distinctive feature of genetic screening is clear: genetic information has implications not only for the individuals who undergo testing, but also for their children, siblings, and parents. The implications of genetic information for family relationships and individuals' feelings concerning these relationships have been discussed frequently by genetic counselors (e.g., Kessler, 1979). Nevertheless, nearly all of the empirical literature concerning the impact of testing reviewed here reports data collected from individual screening participants. Typically, only one member of an immediate family provides psychosocial data to the investigator. When current or potential parents are studied, data are sometimes collected from spouses. The literature clearly shows that family-related issues are paramount in the minds of many screening participants. Nevertheless, we have learned very little about the ways in which family relationships are affected by genetic information. Clinical experience suggests that guilt, shame, resentment, and embarrassment are common emotions experienced by family members affected by genetic diseases or genetic tests. Nance and her colleagues (1991), in a discussion of their HD testing program in Minnesota, noted that "the spouses or companions have been affected as much or more by the genetic diagnosis of HD than have the consultands" (p. 520).

The richness and complexity that characterize these phenomena have not been captured by the many surveys of screening participants. Standardized measures of anxiety or depression simply don't capture the more subtle emotional and relational issues that can be initiated by genetic information. An important exception is the work by Hayden's group concerning HD testing. He and his British Columbia group have reported in-depth case studies, small-scale interview studies, and large-scale prospective studies that illustrate the merit of triangulating different levels of analysis, different measures, and different methods on a complex set of psychosocial issues. Recently, the group proposed a psychological stage model of responses to the diagnosis of HD (Bloch et al., 1993).

One challenge to the justification for genetic screening is the paucity of evidence showing that prenatal genetic information significantly influences parents' decisions concerning affected fetuses (Green, 1990). One of the most striking examples of this comes from the large hemoglobinopathy screening program at the University of Rochester. Rowley et al. (1991a) reported outcomes for 77 pregnancies that were determined through carrier screening to be at high risk for a hemoglobinopathy. The initial screening involved 18,907 women. Of these, 810 had abnormal test results, and the investigators attempted to contact each individual with the permission of her physician. Participants were offered genetic counseling and partner testing. Eighteen amniocenteses were performed, and one pregnancy was terminated.

Rowley et al. (1991a) defend their program on the basis of its demonstrable educational benefits to participants. It is clear that participants in their program were able to make more *informed* decisions, even if they weren't substantially *different* from the decisions they might have made without the genetic information. "Furthermore," as the authors note, "carrier identification may be useful for future reproductive planning, even though some may not apply it to a pregnancy in progress" (p. 445).

Research Needs

Given the large number of studies concerning the psychological aspects of genetic screening, it is surprising that only a narrow range of issues has been investigated. We chose to describe only briefly the extensive literature concerning attitudes toward genetic testing. One of the striking features of that literature is the similarity of questions and methods used. Most investigators report correlations between attitudes or interest and simple demographic variables such as age, sex, number of children, religious affiliation, and education. These data provide some indication (usually an overestimate) of potential utilization of testing. Unfortunately, psychological measures that might provide insight into why members of one demographic group are more interested than members of another are rarely assessed. What is needed now is in-depth, theoretically guided behavioral research.

We need to understand not only why people choose to be tested, but also why two individuals can react so differently to similar information. The assessment of personality and coping styles concerning need for information or need for control may help to explain these individual differences (Miller & Mangan, 1983). Future studies must examine more thoroughly the role of values and beliefs (as opposed to global traits and demographics), as well as the process by which personal health-related experiences (such as the course of the disease in affected family members) shape perceptions of genetic information. The recent work of Tibben and his colleagues (Tibben, Duivenvoorden, et al., 1993; Tibben, Frets, et al., 1993) provides an excellent example of how an examination of moderating variables can enrich our understanding of the individual responses to genetic information.

We also need to know more about those who choose *not* to be tested. Uncertainty reduction appears to be a common motive of individuals who choose to be tested, but the desire to maintain uncertainty and avoid potential distress may be just as important a goal for those who decline testing (Decruyenaere, Evers-Kiebooms, & Van den Berghe, 1993). Because studies of the impact of genetic screening typically exclude those who decline testing, it remains to be seen whether involuntary testing of those who would otherwise decline will produce problems that are not apparent in the current literature.

More data concerning ethnic and cultural differences are needed. Two studies have noted cultural differences in attitudes toward genetic testing (Miller & Schwartz, 1992; Rowley, Loader, Sutera, & Walden, 1987). With the exception of work on sickle cell anemia, most work on psychosocial issues has enlisted primarily white, well-educated study subjects. Given the racial discrimination that resulted from early genetic screening programs for sickle cell anemia (King, 1992), members of ethnic minority groups may be especially reluctant to be tested. Furthermore, the process of recruiting and educating screening participants may have to be tailored to the values and needs of the target ethnic group (Punales-Morejon & Penchaszadeh, 1992).

Just as it cannot be assumed that risk information will produce significant or long-term distress, it cannot be assumed that "good news" is psychologically benign. New information can require psychological adjustment, even when that information reduces an individual's risk of disease. As the research on HD testing has illustrated, individuals who have lived for many years under the cloud of disease threat must consider the possibility that their life perspective and coping skills have been rendered obsolete. When one individual escapes the disease while his or her sibling does not, additional issues arise that can complicate family relationships. These issues have yet to be studied systematically.

CONCLUSION

The research reviewed here demonstrates that significant short-term increases in psychological distress occur among many individuals who are informed of abnormal genetic test results. Given the high false-positive rates of some tests (e.g., MSAFP), it is clear that advocates of screening programs must consider the population impact of screening on the quality of life of screening participants. In contrast, there is little evidence to date that any type of genetic information produces significant increases in global psychological distress in the long term (more than 6 months after test results are communicated).

These conclusions must be qualified by noting some important limitations of the empirical studies discussed here. First, the instruments used in most of these studies were designed to assess global distress of clinical significance. Therefore, they may lack the sensitivity to detect specific concerns or symptoms experienced by screening participants. Second, many studies lack either a no-test control group or an adequate follow-up of individuals who forgo the opportunity to be tested. Much of the evidence reviewed here is based on self-selected screening participants who may not represent those who are most likely to be adversely affected by risk notification. Third, the impact of testing on spouses and other relatives of screening participants has received little attention, even though genetic information is especially relevant to family members (Kessler, 1993). Finally, the large number of studies under way suggests that our understanding of the psychosocial consequences of genetic testing will increase dramatically in the coming decade. Given the tremendous potential of genetic research for improving public health, there is reason to hope that the medical benefits will outweight the potential psychological costs of genetic screening programs.

NOTE

The authors would like to thank Bonnie Baty, Jeff Botkin, Marybeth Hart, Bill McMahon, Jean Nash, and Saara Terry for helpful comments on a draft of the manuscript.

REFERENCES

Amos, C. I., Caporaso, N. E., & Weston, A. (1992). Host factors in lung cancer risk: A review of interdisciplinary studies. *Cancer Epidemiology, Biomarkers & Prevention, 1*, 505–513.

Antley, R. M. (1979). The genetic counselor as facilitator of the counselee's decision process. In A. Capron, M. Lappe, R. F. Murray, Jr., T. Powledge, S. Twiss, & D. Bergsma (Eds.), *Genetic counseling: Facts values and norms* (pp. 137–168). New York: A. R. Liss.

Astbury, J., & Walters, W. A. W. (1979). Amniocentesis in the early second trimester of pregnancy and maternal anxiety. *Australian Family Physician, 8*, 595–599.

Becker, M. H. (Ed.) (1974). The health belief model and personal health behavior. *Health Education Monographs, 2*, 45–50.

Becker, M. H., Kaback, M. M., Rosenstock, I. M., & Ruth, M. V. (1975). Some influences on public participation in a genetic screening program. *Journal of Community Health, 1*, 3–14.

Beeson, D., & Golbus, M. S. (1979). Anxiety engendered by amniocentesis. *Birth Defects: Original Article Series, 15*, 191–197.

Bloch, M., Adam, S., Fuller, A., Kremer, B., Welch, J. P., Wiggins, S., Whyte, P., Huggins, M., Theilmann, J., & Hayden, M. R. (1993). Diagnosis of Huntington disease: A model for the stages of psychological response based on experience of a predictive testing program. *American Journal of Medical Genetics, 47*, 368–374.

Bloch, M., Adam, S., Wiggins, S., Huggins, M., & Hayden, M. R. (1992). Predictive testing for Huntington disease in Canada: The experience of those receiving an increased risk. *American Journal of Medical Genetics, 42*, 499–507.

Bloch, M., Fahy, M., Fox, S., & Hayden, M. R. (1989). Predictive testing for Huntington disease: II. Demographic characteristics, life-style patterns, attitudes, and psychosocial assessments of the first fifty-one test candidates. *American Journal of Medical Genetics, 32*, 217–224.

Botkin, J. R., & Alemagno, S. (1992). Carrier screening for cystic fibrosis: A pilot study of the attitudes of pregnant women. *American Journal of Public Health, 82*(5), 723–725.

Childs, B., Gordis, L., Kaback, M. M., & Kazazian, H. H. (1976). Tay-Sachs screening: Social and psychological impact. *American Journal of Human Genetics, 28*, 550–558.

Cramer, D. W., Harlow, B. L., Willett, W. C., et al. (1989). Galactose consumption and metabolism in relation to the risk for ovarian cancer. *Lancet, 2*, 66–71.

Craufurd, D., Dodge, A., Kerzin-Storrar, L., & Harris, R. (1989). Uptake of presymptomatic predictive testing for Huntington's disease. *Lancet*, 603–605.

Croyle, R. T., & Lerman, C. (1993). Interest in genetic testing for colon cancer susceptibility: Cognitive and emotional correlates. *Preventive Medicine, 22*, 284–292.

Decruyenaere, Evers-Kiebooms, G., & Van den Berghe, H. (1993). Perception of predictive testing for Huntington's disease by young women: preferring uncertainty to certainty? *Medical Genetics, 30*, 557–561.

Di Maio, L., Squitieri, F., Napolitano, G., Campanella, G., Trofatter, J. A., & Conneally, P. M. (1993). Suicide risk in Huntington's disease. *Journal of Medical Genetics, 30*, 293–295.

Evers-Kiebooms, G., Fryns, J., Cassiman, J., & Van den Berghe, H. (Eds.) (1992). *Psychosocial aspects of genetic counseling* (Birth defects: Original article series, Vol. 28, No. 1). New York: Wiley-Liss.

Evers-Kiebooms, G., Swerts, A., & Van den Berghe, H. (1990). Partners of Huntington patients: Implications of the disease and opinions about predictive testing and prenatal diagnosis. *Genetic Counseling, 39*(1), 151–159.

Faden, R. R., Chwalow, A. J., Quaid, K., Chase, G. A., Lopes, C., Leonard, C. O., & Holtzman, N. A. (1987). Prenatal screening and pregnant women's attitudes toward the abortion of defective fetuses. *American Journal of Public Health, 77*, 288–290.

Farrer, L. A. (1986). Suicide and attempted suicide in Huntington disease: Implications for preclinical testing of persons at risk. *American Journal of Medical Genetics, 24*, 305–311.

Fava, G. A., Kellner, R., Michelacci, L., Trombini, G., Pathak, D., Orlandi, C., & Bovicelli, L. (1982). Psychological reactions to amniocentesis: A controlled study. *American Journal of Obstetrics and Gynecology, 143*, 509–513.

Fava, G. A., Trombini, G., Michelacci, L., Linder, J. R., Pathak, D., & Bovicelli, L. (1983). Hostility in women before and after amniocentesis. *Journal of Reproductive Medicine, 28*, 29–34.

Finley, S. C., Varner, P. D., Vinson, P. C., & Finley, W. H. (1977). Participants' reaction to amniocentesis and prenatal genetic studies. *Journal of the American Medical Association, 238*, 2377–2379.

Fisher, L., Rowley, P. T., & Lipkin, M. (1981). Genetic counseling for B-Thalassemia trait following health screening in a health maintenance organization: Comparison of programmed and conventional counseling. *American Journal of Human Genetics, 33*, 987–994.

Fox, S., Bloch, M., Fahy, M., & Hayden, M. R. (1989). Predictive testing for Huntington disease: I. Description of a pilot project in British Columbia. *American Journal of Medical Genetics, 32*, 211–216.

Friend, S. H., Bernards, R., Rojelj, S., et al. (1986). A human DNA segment with properties of the gene that predisposes to retinoblastoma and osteosarcoma. *Nature, 323*, 643–646.

Green, J. M. (1990). *Calming or harming? A critical review of psychological effects of fetal diagnosis on pregnant women.* (Occasional Papers, Second Series No. 2). London: The Galton Institute.

Haynes, R. B., Sackett, D. L., Taylor, D. W., Gibson, E. S., & Johnson, A. L. (1978). Increased absenteeism from work following detection and labelling of hypertensive patients. *New England Journal of Medicine, 299*, 741–744.

Huggins, M., Bloch, M., Wiggins, S., Adam, S., Suchowersky, O., Trew, M., Klimek, M., Greenberg, C. R., Eleff, M., Thompson, L. P., Knight, J., MacLeod, P., Girard, K., Theilman, J., Hedrick, A., & Hayden, M. R. (1992). Predictive testing for Huntington disease in Canada: Adverse effects and unexpected results in those receiving a decreased risk. *American Journal of Medical Genetics, 42*, 508–515.

Jacopini, G. A., D'Amico, R., Frontali, M., & Vivona, G. (1992). Attitudes of persons and their partners toward predictive testing. In G. Evers-Kiebooms et al. (Eds.), *Psychosocial aspects of genetic counseling* (pp. 113–117). New York: Wiley-Liss.

Kessler, S. (Ed.). (1979). *Genetic counselling: Psychological dimensions.* New York: Academic Press.

———. (1989). Psychological aspects of genetic counseling: VI. A critical review of the literature dealing with education and reproduction. *American Journal of Medical Genetics, 34,* 340–353.

———. (1993). Forgotten person in the Huntington disease family. *American Journal of Medical Genetics, 48,* 145–150.

Kessler, S., Field, T., Worth, L., & Mosbarger, H. (1987). Attitudes of persons at risk for Huntington disease toward predictive testing. *American Journal of Medical Genetics, 26,* 259–270.

King, P. A. (1992). The past as prologue: Race, class, and gene discrimination. In G. J. Annas & S. Elias (Eds.), *Gene mapping: Using law and ethics as guides* (pp. 94–111). New York: Oxford University Press.

Lam, R. W., Block, M., Jones, B. D., Marcus, A. M., Fox, S., Amman, W., & Hayden, M. R. (1988). Psychiatric morbidity associated with early clinical diagnosis of Huntington disease in a predictive testing program. *Journal of Clinical Psychiatry, 49*(11), 444–447.

Lerman, C., & Croyle, R. T. (1994). Psychological issues in genetic screening for breast cancer susceptibility. *Archives of Internal Medicine, 154,* 609–616.

Lerman, C., Rimer, B. K., & Engstrom, P. F. (1991). Cancer risk notification: Psychosocial and ethical implications. *Journal of Clinical Oncology, 9*(7), 1275–1282.

Li, F. P., Garber, J. E., Friend, S. H., Strong, L. C., Patenaude, A. F., Juengst, E. T., et al. (1992). Recommendations on predictive testing for germ line p53 mutations among cancer-prone individuals. *Journal of the National Cancer Institute, 84*(15), 1156–1160.

Markel, D. S., Young, A. B., & Penney, J. B. (1987). At-risk persons' attitudes toward presymptomatic and prenatal testing of Huntington disease in Michigan. *American Journal of Medical Genetics, 26,* 295–305.

Marteau, T. M., Johnston, M., Shaw, R. W., Slack, J. (1989). Factors influencing the uptake of screening for open neural-tube defects and amniocentesis to test for Down's syndrome. *British Journal of Obstetrics and Gynecology, 96,* 739–748.

Marteau, T. M., Kidd, J., Cook, R., Johnston, M., Michie, S., Shaw, R. W., & Slack, J. (1988). Screening for Down's syndrome. *British Medical Journal, 279,* 1469.

Marteau, T. M., van Diujn, M., & Ellis, E. (1992). Effects of genetic screening on perceptions of health: A pilot study. *Journal of Medical Genetics, 29,* 24–26.

Massarik, F., & Kaback, M. M. (1981). Genetic disease control: A social psychological approach. Beverly Hills: Sage Publications.

Mastromauro, C., Myers, R. H., & Berkman, B. (1987). Attitudes toward presymptomatic testing in Huntington disease. *American Journal of Medical Genetics, 26,* 271–282.

McNair, D. M., Lorr, M., & Droppleman, L. F. (1971). *Profile of Mood States Manual.* San Diego: Educational & Industrial Testing Service.

Meissen, G. J., & Berchek, R. L. (1987). Intended use of predictive testing by those at risk for Huntington disease. *American Journal of Medical Genetics, 26,* 283–293.

Mennie, M. E., Gilfillan, A., Compton, M., Curtis, L., Liston, W. A., Pullen, I., Whyte, D. A., & Brock, D. J. H. (1992). Prenatal screening for cystic fibrosis. *Lancet, 340,* 214–216.

Miller, S. M. (1980). When is a little knowledge a dangerous thing? Coping with stressful events by monitoring versus blunting. In S. Levine & H. Ursin

(Eds.), *Coping and Health: Proceedings of a NATO Conference* (pp. 145–169). New York: Plenum Press.

Miller, S. M., & Mangan, C. E. (1983). Interacting effects of information and coping style in adapting to gynecologic distress: Should the doctor tell all? *Journal of Personality and Social Psychology, 45,* 223–236.

Miller, S. R., & Schwartz, R. H. (1992). Attitudes toward genetic testing of Amish, Mennonite, and Hutterite families with cystic fibrosis. *American Journal of Public Health, 82,* 236–242.

Milunsky, A. (1975). Risk of amniocentesis for prenatal diagnosis. *New England Journal of Medicine, 293,* 932–933.

Nance, M. A., Leroy, B. S., Orr, H. T., Parker, T., Rich, S. S., & Heston, L. L. (1991). Protocol for genetic testing in Huntington disease: Three years of experience in Minnesota. *American Journal of Medical Genetics, 40,* 518–522.

Phipps, S., & Zinn, A. B. (1986a). Psychological response to amniocentesis: I. Mood state and adaptation to pregnancy. *American Journal of Medical Genetics, 25,* 131–142.

———. (1986b). Psychological response to amniocentesis: II. Effects of coping style. *American Journal of Medical Genetics, 25,* 143–148.

Punales-Morejon, D., & Penchaszadeh, V. B. (1992). Psychosocial aspects of genetic counseling: Cross-cultural issues. G. Evers-Kiebooms, et al. (Eds.), *Psychosocial aspects of genetic counseling* (pp. 11–15). New York: Wiley-Liss.

Quaid, K. A., Brandt, J., Faden, R. R., & Folstein, S. E. (1989). Knowledge, attitude and the decision to be tested for Huntington's disease. *Clinical Genetics, 36,* 431–438.

Quaid, K. A., & Morris, M. (1993). Reluctance to undergo predictive testing: The case of Huntington disease. *American Journal of Medical Genetics, 45,* 41–45.

Reading, A. E. (1983). The influence of maternal anxiety on the course and outcome of pregnancy: A review. *Health Psychology, 2,* 187–202.

Robinson, J. O., Hibbard, B. M., & Laurence, K. M. (1984). Anxiety during a crisis: Emotional effects of screening for neural tube defects. *Journal of Psychosomatic Research, 28*(2), 163–169.

Rowley, P. T., Fisher, L., & Lipkin, M. (1979). Screening and genetic counseling for B-Thalassemia trait in a population unselected for interest: Effects on knowledge and mood. *American Journal of Human Genetics, 31,* 718–730.

———. (1984). Screening and genetic counseling for Beta-Thalassemia trait in a population unselected for interest: Comparison of three counseling methods. *American Journal of Human Genetics, 36,* 677–689.

Rowley, P. T., Loader, S. O., Sutera, C. J., & Walden, M. (1987). Prenatal hemoglobinopathy screening: Receptivity of Southeast Asian refugees. *American Journal of Preventive Medicine, 3,* 317–322.

Rowley, P. T., Loader, S. O., Sutera, C. J., Walden, M., & Kozyra, A. (1991a). Prenatal screening for hemoglobinopathies. I. A prospective regional trial. *American Journal of Human Genetics, 48,* 439–446.

———. (1991b). Prenatal screening for hemoglobinopathies. III. Applicability of the health belief model. *American Journal of Human Genetics, 48,* 452–459.

Shapiro, D. A., & Shapiro, L. R. (1989). Pitfalls in Tay-Sachs carrier detection: Physician referral patterns and patient ignorance. *New York State Journal of Medicine, 89,* 317–319.

Smith, R. A., Williams, D. K., Sibert, J. R., & Harper, P. S. (1990). Attitudes of mothers to neonatal screening for Duchenne muscular dystrophy. *British Medical Journal, 300,* 1112.

Spielberger, C. D., Gorsuch, R. L., & Lushene, R. E. (1970). *Manual for the State-Trait Anxiety Inventory.* Palo Alto,California: Consulting Psychologists Press.

Spurdle, A., Kromberg, J., Rosendorff, J., & Jenkins, T. (1991). Prenatal diagnosis for Huntington's disease: A molecular and psychological study. *Prenatal Diagnosis, 11,* 177–185.

Stamatoyannopoulos, G. (1974). Problems of screening and counseling in the hemoglobinopathies. In A. G. Motulsky & W. Lenz (Eds.), *Birth defects: Proceedings of the Fourth International Conference, Vienna, 1973.* Geneva: Excerpta Medica.

Sujansky, E., Kreutzer, S. B., Johnson, A. M., Lezotte, D. C., Schrier, R. W., & Gabow, P. A. (1990). Attitudes of at-risk and affected individuals regarding presymptomatic testing for autosomal dominant polycystic kidney disease. *American Journal of Medical Genetics, 35*(4), 510–515.

Tabor, A., & Jonsson, M. H. (1987). Psychological impact of amniocentesis in low risk women. *Prenatal Diagnosis, 7,* 443–449.

Thompson, M. W., McInnes, R. R., & Willard, H. F. (1991). *Genetics in Medicine* (5th ed.). Philadelphia: W. B. Saunders & Co.

Tibben, A., Duivenvoorden, H. J., Vegter-van der Vlis, M., Niermeijer, M. F., Frets, P. G., van de Kamp, J. J. P., Roos, R. A. C., Rooijmans, H. G. M., & Verhage, F. (1993). Presymptomatic DNA testing for Huntington disease: Identifying the need for psychological intervention. *American Journal of Medical Genetics, 48,* 137–144.

Tibben, A., Frets, P. G., van de Kamp, J. J. P., Niermeijer, M. F., Vegter-van der Vlis, M., Roos, R. A. C., van Ommen, G. B., Duivenvoorden, H. J., & Verhage, F. (1993). Presymptomatic DNA-testing for Huntington disease: Pretest attitudes and expectations of applicants and their partners in the Dutch program. *American Journal of Medical Genetics, 48,* 10–16.

Tyler, A., & Morris, M. (1990). National symposium on problems of presymptomatic testing for Huntington's disease, Cardiff. *Journal of Medical Ethics, 16,* 41–42.

Tyler, A., Quarrell, O. W. J., Lazarov, L. P., Meredith, A. L., & Harper, B. S. (1990). Exclusion testing in pregnancy for Huntington's disease. *Journal of Medical Genetics, 27*(8), 488–495.

Vineis, P., Caporaso, N., Tannenbaum, S. R., et al. (1990). Acetylation phenotype, carcinogen-hemoglobin adducts, and cigarette smoking. *Cancer Research, 50,* 3002–3004.

Vogelstein, B., Fearon, E. R., Hamilton, S. R., et al. (1988). Genetic alterations during colorectal tumor development. *New England Journal of Medicine, 319,* 525–532.

Watson, E. K., Mayall, E., Chapple, J., Dalziel, M., Harrington, K., Williams, C., & Williamson, R. (1991). Screening for carriers of cystic fibrosis through primary care health services. *British Medical Journal, 303:* 504–507.

Watson, E. K., Mayall, E. S., Lamb, J., Chapple, J., & Williamson, R. (1992). Psychological and social consequences of community carrier screening programme for cystic fibrosis. *The Lancet, 340,* 217–220.

Weinberg, R. A. (1991). Tumor suppressor genes. *Science, 254,* 1138–1146.

Wertz, D. C., Janes, S. R., Rosenfield, J. M., & Erbe, R. W. (1992). Attitudes toward the prenatal diagnosis of cystic fibrosis: Factors in decision making among affected families. *American Journal of Human Genetics, 50*, 1077–1085.

Wexler, N. (1991). Presymptomatic testing for Huntington's disease: Harbinger of the new genetics. In Z. Bankowski & A. M. Capron (Eds.), *Genetics, ethics, and human values: Human genome mapping, genetic screening, and gene therapy* (pp. 80–92). Geneva: Council for International Organizations of Medical Sciences.

Wiggins, S., Whyte, P., Huggins, M., Adam, S., Theilman, J., Block, M., Sheps, S. B., Schechter, M. T., & Hayden, M. R. (1992). The psychological consequences of predictive testing for Huntington's disease. *New England Journal of Medicine, 327*, 1401–1405.

Wooldridge, E. Q., & Murray, Jr., R. F. (1988). The health orientation scale: a measure of feelings about sickle cell trait. *Social Biology, 35*(1–2), 123–136.

3

Psychosocial Impact of Cholesterol Screening and Management

KAREN GLANZ
MARY BETH GILBOY

Elevated blood cholesterol is a major risk factor for coronary heart disease (CHD) and a significant public health problem. This highly prevalent, asymptomatic risk factor affects one fifth to one half of all American adults (Sempos et al., 1993) and can usually be prevented or controlled once it is identified. Although mean total cholesterol levels in U.S. adults aged 20 to 74 have consistently declined between 1960 and 1991, an estimated 52 million Americans, or 29% of all adults, have levels that warrant dietary change and 7% are candidates for drug therapy (Johnson et al., 1993; Sempos et al., 1993).

Identification of individuals with elevated blood cholesterol (BC) levels* is the first step toward reducing CHD risk through cholesterol management. After screening, individuals with elevated levels should be referred to physicians for further diagnostic evaluation and appropriate treatment. The primary treatment approach is dietary change; medication (along with diet) is indicated if cholesterol reduction cannot be achieved by dietary means alone (Expert Panel, 1993).

There are two major types of detection strategies for identifying individuals with elevated cholesterol: case finding in medical (clinical)

---

*Unless otherwise indicated, the term "cholesterol level" as used in this chapter refers to blood cholesterol level. The term "serum cholesterol level" reflects a common method for measuring blood cholesterol. Levels can also be measured on plasma with results multiplied by 1.03 to arrive at the serum equivalent (Report of the Expert Panel, 1988).

settings and screening in other locations such as worksites, shopping malls, and churches (Ernst & Cleeman, 1988; Expert Panel, 1993). The National Cholesterol Education Program (NCEP) recommends routine cholesterol testing in all medical contacts, i.e., case finding, but has not endorsed widespread community-based screening (Expert Panel, 1993). However, numerous reports of public screening and education have been published, in addition to the three large community trials of public screening funded by the National Heart, Lung, and Blood Institute (NHLBI) (Havas, Greenland, Wones, & Schucker, 1989). Further, a population-based approach to cholesterol reduction based on adoption of low-fat dietary change and avoidance of overweight has been advised (NCEP Population Panel, 1990). The dietary recommendations for primary prevention are, in fact, identical to the initial treatment guidelines for people with elevated cholesterol levels.

With the widespread use of cholesterol screening (terminology used here to subsume both clinical case finding and public screening), concerns have been raised about the relative benefits and risks of mass cholesterol-control efforts (Glanz, 1990). The primary debate has centered on the disease control effects of cholesterol-lowering interventions, with arguments either noting significant benefits in delaying CHD onset and increasing life expectancy (Gotto et al., 1990; Grover et al., 1992) or contending that the safety of cholesterol-lowering strategies has not been proven (Muldoon & Manuck, 1992; Jacobs et al., 1993). A second type of debate concerns the possible negative societal and personal consequences of screening: high consumption of limited health care resources (Pearson, Bowlin, & Sigmund, 1990; Kinlay, 1988) and psychological distress induced by labeling asymptomatic individuals as "sick" (Lefebvre, Hursey, & Carleton, 1988; Hulley & Newman, 1992), as well as the possibility of false reassurance, inadequate technology, lack of sufficient trained personnel, and poor adherence with therapeutic regimens (NCEP, 1987; Glanz, 1990).

In this chapter, we review the literature on the psychological and behavioral impact of screening programs for high blood cholesterol in adults. First, we review factors affecting contemporary cholesterol screening and management, including technology, trends in screening and treatment, and accepted standards for programs of screening, education and counseling. Next, we review studies reporting on the impact of cholesterol screening, notification, and education in four areas: psychological distress, awareness and knowledge, referral for follow-up, and behavior change/risk factor reduction. Methodological issues, future research needs, and implications of these findings for future cholesterol-screening programs will also be discussed.

Publications were identified through government sources, a search of the MEDLINE bibliographic database, and backward searches of reference lists in published articles and reports. Most sources used here were published after the 1985 Consensus Conference and the majority are less than 5 years old. For studies assessing the impact of cholesterol screening, only those studies in which participants or subjects received feedback about their cholesterol level and risk status after screening are included.

FACTORS AFFECTING CHOLESTEROL SCREENING AND MANAGEMENT

Cholesterol screening and management activities occur within the context of public health and medical policy and practice as well as rapidly changing technology. These contextual factors influence the perceptions and behaviors of individuals who receive screening. This section discusses the state of screening technology and related issues, trends and determinants of cholesterol screening and management, and state of the art guidelines for cholesterol screening programs.

Screening Technology

Cholesterol screening requires analysis of blood samples using special-ized instrumentation, either in a clinical laboratory (usually by veni-puncture) or with a portable blood cholesterol analyzer (usually by fingerstick). The development of portable instruments has been central to the widespread dissemination of cholesterol screening, especially in public settings. These "desktop analyzers" are distinguished by their portability, rapid analysis, and ability to provide immediate feedback to screenees. They also enable individual physicians' offices to complete initial cholesterol assessments without depending on out-side laboratories.

To promote accurate and precise cholesterol measurements, strict performance standards were established for clinical laboratories, call-ing for intralab variation of less than 3% to 5% (U.S. Department of Health and Human Services [USDHHS], 1987). Similar guidelines and recommendations for quality assurance and consideration of biologic sources of variability were released for clinical use of desktop ana-lyzers (USDHHS, 1990). Systematic evaluations of several portable cholesterol analyzers used in a clinical setting according to manufacturers' recommended procedures found them to perform with good precision and accuracy when compared with standardized laboratories (Koch, Hassemer, Wiebe, & Laessig, 1988; Burke & Fischer, 1988). However, evaluations of various portable cholesterol analyzers in public settings found significant inaccuracies (Naughton, Luepker, & Strickland, 1990; Stave, Winslow, & Conner, 1991; Havas, Bishop, Koumijian, Reisman, & Wozenski, 1992). Fingerstick methods tended to underestimate laboratory cholesterol values (Naughton et al., 1990; Lasater, Lefebvre, Assaf, Saritelli, & Carleton, 1987), instruments malfunctioned in the field (Havas, Bishop, et al., 1992), and a significant number of participants were misclassified, mainly into "false negative" risk categories (Lasater et al., 1987; Naughton et al., 1990; Havas, Bishop, et al., 1992).

Guidelines for cholesterol screening advise that a diagnosis of elevated blood cholesterol should be based on repeat measurements (at different times) along with an overall risk assessment (Gwynne, 1991; Expert Panel, 1988 and 1993), as at least two specimens are needed to estimate a true "total" cholesterol with 95% confidence (Cooper, Myers, Smith, & Schlant, 1992). More detailed lipid analysis is also necessary (Expert Panel, 1988 and 1993). In addition, training and quality control are essential, particularly in public settings (Boyle, Lenhert, Porter, & Pryor, 1992; Naughton et al., 1990; Havas, Bishop et al., 1992).

Little research has addressed the implications of analytical accuracy for education and feedback to screenees. One investigator concluded by recommending "routine use of confidence intervals when discussing cholesterol measurements with patients" (Stave et al., 1991), an interesting suggestion that might create confusion and/or arouse a *lack of confidence* in the results. Despite widespread media coverage of the unreliability of cholesterol (and other laboratory) tests, we found only one study that evaluated subjects' ratings of the accuracy of cholesterol measurements. In an experiment on screening feedback with undergraduate university students, Croyle, Sun, and Louie (1993) found that borderline-high subjects rated tests as less accurate than did desirable-level feedback subjects. Considering this finding along with the tendency of portable instruments to *underestimate* cholesterol values, it is possible that many participants in cholesterol screening are either falsely reassured (due to technology failure) or minimizing the threat of a serious risk factor (due to psychological processes). These possible consequences merit further evaluation with diverse population segments as the technology spreads.

Trends in Cholesterol Control Activities

The past decade has brought a dramatic increase in interest and activity related to cholesterol reduction. This has been marked by two major occurrences: the development of scientific consensus (Consensus Conference, 1985) and the establishment of the National Cholesterol Education Program (NCEP) by the National Heart, Lung, and Blood Institute (NHLBI) in 1985. The NCEP is a government-coordinated, intersectoral effort to improve professional and public knowledge, awareness, and behavior related to cholesterol through improved detection, diagnosis, and treatment of high blood cholesterol levels (Ernst & Cleeman, 1988). The first activities of the NCEP were aimed at promoting detection of high blood cholesterol in all adults age 20 and over, and further evaluation and treatment for those with elevated levels (Report of the NCEP Expert Panel, 1988). Although the ultimate goal of screening is to identify high-risk individuals, it also provides a channel for nutrition education and CHD prevention awareness, aims that are central to a public health approach to cholesterol control.

Participation in Screening. Since the inception of the NCEP, numerous screening programs have been established. According to the Cholesterol Awareness Survey, a national cross-sectional sample survey (in 1983, 1986, and 1990), an estimated 65% of American adults had their cholesterol checked by 1990, a 20% increase over 1986 (Schucker et al., 1991). Analyses of responses to the Centers for Disease Control (CDC)'s Behavioral Risk Factor Surveillance System (BRFSS) survey in 1989 and 1990 yielded similar findings, with state medians at 56% and 63%, respectively (CDC, 1990; 1992). Screening is more common among older adults, whites, well-educated groups (CDC, 1990; Polednak, 1992), and those who report more physician visits and regular checkups (Polednak, 1992; Hyman, Simons-Morton, Ho, Dunn, & Rubovitz, 1993). Low-income individuals, blacks, Hispanics, men, and younger adults are underrepresented at public screenings (Havas, Koumjian, Reisman, Hsu, & Wozenski, 1991; Hyman, Paradis, & Flora, 1992; Hyman, Simons-Morton, et al., 1993). However, in site-specific screenings, such as worksites and churches, participants do not differ significantly from the overall populations at those locations (Wilson & Edmunson, 1991; Gans, Lefebvre et al., 1989; Hyman et al., 1992).

Cholesterol Awareness and Knowledge. Both public and professional awareness about cholesterol as a risk factor for cardiovascular disease have increased since the early 1980s (Schucker et al., 1987; Schucker et al., 1991). Nearly all adults have heard about cholesterol, though minorities are somewhat less aware (Sprafka, Burke, Folsom, & Hahn, 1989). Recent surveys found that awareness ranged from 76% in a low-income, urban population (Hyman, Simons-Morton, et al., 1993) to 90% in two predominantly white, suburban samples (Polednak, 1992). Interest and information seeking about nutrition to reduce CHD risk are very high throughout the general public (FMI, 1992; Hyman, Simons-Morton, et al., 1993).

Surveys that have inquired about screenees' reported knowledge of their cholesterol levels also show increases in recent years (Shucker et al., 1991), with BRFSS data indicating an increase in the median from 23% to 29% between 1989 and 1990 (CDC, 1990, 1992). However, these data should be interpreted with caution; the national surveys were conducted by telephone and did not permit verification that "known" levels were accurate. In fact, in one study that compared patient reports to values recorded in medical records, all of the patients could accurately state their risk status but fewer than half accurately remembered their exact cholesterol number (Glanz et al., 1990).

Trend analysis of both national and regional surveys has demonstrated consistent increases in cholesterol-related knowledge, defined as knowledge of risk factor relationships and dietary recommendations, over the past decade (Schucker et al., 1991; Frank, Winkleby, Fortmann, Rockhill, & Farquhar, 1992; Frank, Winkleby, Fortmann, & Farquhar, 1993). However, the Health and Diet Surveys, sponsored by the U.S. Food and Drug Administration (FDA) and the NHLBI in 1983, 1986, and 1988, revealed poor levels of knowledge related to dietary fat and cholesterol and only modest improvements on selected items (Levy, Fein, & Stephenson, 1993). The discrepancy between these surveys and those mentioned above lies in the difficulty of the questions: the FDA/NHLBI surveys asked nutrient-specific, difficult questions (e.g., "which foods are low in polyunsaturated vs. saturated fat?") whereas the others asked more general questions about CVD risk factors and dietary practices. The different conceptualizations of "cholesterol-related knowledge" as they apply to the general public appear to account for the discrepant findings and raise concerns about the construct validity of the survey measures (Axelson & Brinberg, 1992).

Dietary Behavior Change. A substantial minority of respondents to national surveys (Schucker et al., 1991) and surveys in California (Frank et al., 1992) and Texas (Hyman et al., 1993) report improved dietary practices to prevent or control elevated blood cholesterol. Although these survey measures used only limited assessments of eating patterns, in at least one study they were associated with actual reductions in cholesterol levels (Frank et al., 1992). These data suggest that media messages associated with cholesterol control activities are also affecting behavior in nonclinical populations.

Physician and Health System Factors. In the United States, guidelines for cholesterol screening and management place the majority of activity within a physician-led health care setting (Gotto et al., 1990; Expert Panel, 1993). And although there is increased awareness among health professionals that high blood cholesterol (HBC) is an important and treatable risk for CHD (Schucker et al., 1991), physicians' detection and treatment practice patterns are not consistent with established guidelines (Glanz & Gilboy, 1992; Maiman, Greenland, Hildreth, & Cox, 1991). Studies of both inpatients and outpatients that used chart audits showed wide variations in physician practices of recognizing elevated cholesterol, ordering full lipid profiles, physician counseling, prescribing dietary change and drugs, and referral for further counseling. Despite the varied study populations, all these studies indicated substantial discrepancies between guidelines for clinical management of elevated cholesterol and actual practices (Glanz & Gilboy, 1992).

In another report, analysis of BRFSS responses from 154,735 adults in 37 states regarding identification and treatment of HBC revealed that the percentage of those who are being treated is less than one third of those who need treatment (Giles et al., 1993). While this probably reflects some patient nonadherence with referral advice, it no doubt reflects physicians' actions and system factors as well. In addition, there are financial barriers to clinical management of HBC that are of concern. These include lack of reimbursement for outpatient nutrition counseling and for time with nonphysician health educators (Glanz, 1988).

Guidelines for Screening, Education, Advice, and Counseling

Contemporary guidelines for cholesterol screening and management strongly urge screening providers to offer feedback, education, and follow-up. Many lessons learned in hypertension control programs in the 1970s and 1980s were important foundations for cholesterol screening guidelines (Harlan & Stross, 1985; Lefebvre et al., 1988). The guidelines that have been promulgated are intended both to maximize the benefits of screening and to mitigate or minimize any negative consequences. They include avoiding definitive diagnostic labels and noting that more than one measure is needed for conclusive evaluation; making specific referrals for further evaluation; following up on participants; assessing dietary behaviors as a basis for providing specific advice to change; making specific positive behavioral recommendations; and engaging participants in active problem solving and goal setting (Lefebvre, Linnan, Sundaram, & Ronan, 1990).

Most of the cholesterol screening studies we identified contained statements about the inclusion of strategies based on these guidelines. Thus, with the exception of a few laboratory-based studies, it is not really possible to distinguish the screening process from the subsequent "intervention" that consists of feedback, education, advice, and referral. Also, many articles give insufficient details on the content or format of the educational components. Because of these blurred distinctions, nearly all the investigations reported here are assumed to have some type of "management" (feedback, education, advice, referral) component. Where various specific approaches were evaluated in experiments, or where details were provided, we so indicate.

IMPACT OF CHOLESTEROL SCREENING, NOTIFICATION, AND EDUCATION

Increasingly, studies are being reported that investigate the impact of screening, notification, and education for the control of high blood cholesterol. The general series of steps for cholesterol reduction involves detection/awareness, successful referral for evaluation, adherence to a recommended therapeutic regimen (diet or drugs), and risk factor reduction. Although these steps are analogous to steps for high blood pressure control (Glanz & Scholl, 1982), the sequence may differ, largely because the primary treatment modality for HBC is dietary change. To manage high cholesterol, dietary change can occur *without* completing referral and evaluation by a physician (Glanz, 1988). In addition, because control of high blood pressure usually requires long-term medication, the recognition of an "illness" state may be more likely than for HBC. Nevertheless, both HBC and high blood pressure are serious, asymptomatic risk factors for CHD and require long-term behavior changes for their control (Harlan & Stross, 1985). Thus, our examination of the impact of cholesterol screening and follow-up addresses four types of outcomes: labeling or psychological distress in response to detection of elevated levels; memory awareness, and knowledge; referral for follow-up evaluation and treatment; and behavior change and cholesterol reduction.

Labeling and Psychological Distress

Concern about the possible negative effects of participation in cholesterol screening programs derives from some studies in the 1970s that showed that individuals manifested psychological and behavioral symptoms after being told that they had high blood pressure. They were found to identify themselves as "sick," experience psychological distress, rate themselves as in poorer health, and have increased absenteeism from work (MacDonald, Sackett, Haynes, & Taylor, 1984). Several investigations of cholesterol detection and treatment examined this concern. Brett (1991) reported on six case studies in which each patient experienced distress, psychosomatic symptoms, increased anxiety, or problems with medication. Although the case findings have limited generalizability, Brett recommended research on larger patient populations to examine the consequences of new diagnosis and treatment for HBC.

Tymstra and Bieleman (1987) surveyed 267 men who attended a cholesterol screening in a small town in the Netherlands and found that 23% of participants had abnormal results, with 19% of these reporting surprise and 8% (or five men) stating that they were shocked by the results and had become "anxious and uncertain." By contrast, 44% of those receiving a "healthy" report stated that they did not have to change their (unhealthy) lifestyles because they were healthy. Thus, out of the total sample, a very small percentage reported distress and a significant minority experienced some false reassurance to justify unhealthy behavior (Tymstra & Bieleman, 1987).

Fischer, Guinan, Burke, Karp, and Richards (1990) administered a mailed questionnaire that included items on perceived general health and psychosocial well-being (from the General Well-Being Schedule) to one third of all adults who participated in a screening program at a shopping mall in Georgia. Using a 5-point Likert-type measure of "disturbance," they found increased levels of disturbance as cholesterol levels increased (desirable BC = mean of 1.7, high BC = mean of 4.0). They also found significantly lower general health scores with higher cholesterol levels but no significant difference in absenteeism among risk groups. Limitations of this study included the lack of baseline measures and possible response bias (with only a 62% response rate).

Three studies of cholesterol screening used designs that were more rigorous, incorporating baseline measures and/or comparison groups. In the Massachusetts Model Systems for Blood Cholesterol Screening Project, Havas, Reisman, Hsu, and Koumjian (1991) administered a baseline questionnaire to 3,489 participants before screening, education, and referral. They readministered the questionnaire to screenees categorized as having high blood cholesterol, obtaining an 82% completion rate. The questionnaire included nine questions on health perceptions from the Rand Corporation's General Health Perceptions Questionnaire. The combined scores of the entire sample showed significant *positive* changes at follow-up, with one item about "feeling good" decreasing in older participants; thus, their data do not provide any evidence of negative effects of screening.

At baseline and after initial and follow-up cholesterol screenings for volunteers in a California community, Hyman, Flora, Reynolds, Johannson, and Farquhar (1991) administered a quality of life instrument to 184 adults. They found no adverse impact of the screening and education process for those with either elevated or normal BC levels on either subjective health status, missed work days, or restricted activity days.

In a prospective study of worksite-based cholesterol screening in Sweden, Rastam, Frick, and Gullberg (1991) examined whether being informed of high blood cholesterol would induce feelings of ill health, reflected in increased work absenteeism. They provided screening for 1,594 male construction workers; those who were initially found to have HBC were invited to be rescreened, and received nonthreatening information and advice about positive action steps. Using insurance data from before and after the screening, the number of sick days and sick leave episodes were recorded. The chances that hypercholesterolemic men would increase the number of sick days or of sick episodes was no more than for normocholesterolemic men. The investigators concluded that if people know that they have HBC, it does not necessarily mean they perceive themselves as really ill.

The limited data on responses to cholesterol screening, particularly the three studies with designs that permitted ruling out alternative explanations, suggest that overall psychological well-being is not adversely affected by a diagnosis of high blood cholesterol. These findings may be due in part to the type of feedback and its delivery used in the controlled studies, because earlier studies of risk factor screening indicated that negative effects can be prevented or alleviated with clear information given in a sympathetic and supportive manner (MacDonald et al., 1984). However, it is also possible that the broad measures that were used are insensitive to some kinds of worry, disruption, and stress induced by risk notification (Lerman et al., 1991).

It is further important to note that these investigations shed little light on the coping processes used by newly diagnosed individuals with HBC. In both laboratory and community settings, Croyle et al.

(1993) found that people receiving a diagnosis of borderline-high cholesterol engaged in threat minimization, viewing HBC as more common and as a less serious threat to health than did individuals who
were given desirable readings. While the Croyle et al. studies did not
reflect "usual practice" of providing tentative risk level information
(that states the need for repeat measurements) and supportive, specific
advice, they suggest that the cognitive processes of health appraisal
may not have been observable in the studies described earlier.

Memory, Awareness, and Knowledge

Three articles report on patients' memory, awareness, and knowledge
about their cholesterol screening and management experience after
being found to have HBC and receiving medical treatment. Kinlay
and Heller (1990) surveyed 552 patients from general medical practices
in Australia and found that those with borderline-high BC levels were
significantly less likely to recall receiving a recommendation about
the need for cholesterol reduction and less likely to recall receiving
dietary advice, than those with high BC levels. The finding that patients
with borderline-high levels more often "forgot" their diagnosis and
the doctor's advice is consistent with the findings of Croyle et al.
(1993) regarding threat minimization as a coping strategy.

Two reports of telephone surveys of patients who had received
diagnosis and counseling during different phases of a physician-based
nutrition program in Minnesota examined patients' perceptions about
cholesterol, heart disease, their own risk status, and services they
received. In both surveys, respondents were predominantly white,
aged 53, and had more than a high school education. Glanz et al. (1990)
conducted telephone interviews with 94 patients who had received
cholesterol counseling and compared the response with clinic records.
More than 95% of the respondents knew they had high cholesterol
and could explain why it was an important health problem. However,
only 43.8% of those with recorded cholesterol values could state the
correct level. Higher numbers were given by 7.4%, lower numbers
were given by 8.5%, and another 32.8% said they could not remember
the number. There was no significant relationship between the time
between the visit and the interview and whether the patient correctly
remembered the cholesterol level. In addition, a substantial proportion
of the patients did not recall receiving advice from a physician or
discussing specific behavioral goals with the counselor (a dietitian or
nurse), though 98% remembered receiving print educational materials.

Allen, Bache-Wiig, and Hunninghake (1992) reported on interviews with 179 primary care clinic patients in a later phase of the same study. Ninety-eight percent of the patients correctly stated that they had borderline-high or high cholesterol levels, and 94% could give a plausible numerical level. The numbers matched the reported risk level category 85% of the time. However, these numbers were not compared with recorded chart values so it is not possible to determine whether they were in fact accurate. Ninety-seven percent of the patients could give one valid reason why cholesterol was important to their health, and 88% could state specific dietary recommendations for lowering their cholesterol levels.

These studies provide a mixed picture of patients' memory for information related to their diagnosis and treatment for high blood cholesterol. All three investigations are limited to patients who have received follow-up treatment, and are thus *more* likely to be motivated and involved in risk reduction than those who do not follow through on referrals (see the next section). They found high rates of remembering a general diagnosis, its importance, and the type of behavior changes recommended. However, memory of specific cholesterol levels and of individual components of counseling were often faulty. These findings can be interpreted in several ways. On the one hand, recall of a specific cholesterol number may not be a prerequisite for action, and thus a poor indicator of "knowledge" about the condition. Alternatively, patient misunderstanding and memory failure are common in patient counseling (Ley, 1987), and these findings may simply reflect typical situations. A further possibility is that compromised memory is the result of coping responses to stressful information. The research to date in this area is limited and further studies should use appropriate comparison groups and address the association between recall of various aspects of patients' situations and subsequent compliance and risk reduction.

Referral for Follow-Up

After detection of elevated cholesterol levels through screening, follow-up referral adherence is important for further evaluation and/or treatment and counseling by a health professional. However, many individuals who are informed that their BC levels are above desirable levels do not adhere with referral advice. Table 3-1 summarizes studies that examined follow-up referral adherence rates for a wide variety of populations.

Seven studies are primarily descriptive and did not test specific interventions. These studies found follow-up rates ranging from a low of 21% to a high of 81%, with a median at about 50%. One noteworthy finding in several of the studies was that follow-up adherence was higher for individuals classified as "high" than for those with "borderline high" levels (Fischer et al., 1990; Gordon, Klag, & Whelton, 1990; Gans, Lasater, Linnan, LaPane, & Carleton, 1990). The exception to this was a study of follow-up to public screening in California, in which follow-up rates were 34% among those with *desirable* BC levels and 32%, or slightly lower, among those with high BC at the screening (Hyman et al., 1991). Analysis of Rhode Island data by Gans et al. (1990) showed that the difference in follow-up rates between high and borderline-high screenees occurred only among younger adults and not for those over age 65.

Of the four intervention studies, two found no significant impact of special follow-up interventions (Fitzgerald, Gibbons, & Agnew, 1991; Owen, James, Henriksen, & van Beurden, 1990). However, Fitzgerald et al. (1991) observed significantly higher adherence for subjects with high BC compared to those with borderline BC (44% vs. 17%). Havas et al. (1991) found that reminder postcards resulted in higher follow-through rates but that other factors associated with better follow-up included higher education levels, prior history of high cholesterol, higher BC levels, and older age. Maiman, Hildreth, Cox, and Greenland (1992) found no difference with either a professional or lay communicator but found that reminder letters and coupon offers yielded higher follow-up among individuals with no prior awareness of their elevated BC.

These studies suggest that many factors influence follow-up adherence rates, and that in some cases special postscreening interventions can improve follow-up success. They also suggest that older individuals, those with higher BC levels, and those with more education are more likely to seek further evaluation and/or treatment. Risk level seems to be the most consistent correlate of follow-up adherence. The contradictory findings of Havas, Koumjian, et al. (1991) and Maiman et al. (1992) raise the question of how "previous history" or prior awareness of elevated cholesterol affects interpretation of screening results and subsequent actions to seek evaluation and/or treatment.

Behavior Change and Cholesterol Reduction

Many studies have included assessments of changes in dietary behavior to achieve cholesterol reduction and of decreased cholesterol levels following screening and counseling. In these studies, change in BC levels can be regarded as a proxy measure of adherence to behavioral

Table 3.1. Follow-Up Referral Adherence for Elevated Blood Cholesterol

Citation	Sample	Type of Screening and Advice	Special Intervention(s)	Adherence Rate	Comments
Rastam, Luepker, & Pirie (1988)	424 adults w/high BC levels after 2 measures	Public screening	—	57%	
Fischer et al. (1990)	1,089 adults	Public screening at mall	—	68.0% of those classified as high 30.5% of those classified as borderline-high	Follow-up (FU) = re-test and discuss w/MD
Tymstra & Bieleman (1987)	107 men in the Netherlands w/ elevated BC	Mass screening for CVD risk factors	—	82%	Follow-up = saw MD or dietician
Gordon et al. (1990)	375 adults in Baltimore	Medical clinic and shopping mall screenings	—	50% of those classified as high 22% of those classified as borderline-high	Higher adherence for high levels than borderline
Gans et al. (1990)	137 older (65+ yrs.) and younger (18–64 yrs.) adults in Rhode Island	SCORE (screening and referral events) at various locations	—	50% of those classified as high 21% of those classified as borderline-high	No difference between high and borderline rates among *older* adults
Hyman et al. (1991)	188 adults in California	Public screening with printed information on BC level, booklets, and referral for those with HBC	—	32% with high BC 34% with desirable BC levels	Possibly biased due to use of volunteer sample
Burns et al. (1991)	100 adults with HBC levels	Screening in emergency room while there for non-BC reasons	—	53%	

Author (year)	Population	Setting	Intervention	Results	Findings
Fitzgerald et al. (1991)	268 employees with elevated BC levels	Follow-up to a worksite screening program	Booster mailing with personal letter, advice, and NCEP pamphlet / No-intervention control (randomized)	44% for high BC / 17% for borderline BC	No difference due to booster mailing intervention
Havas Koumjian et al. (1991)	2,627 adults with HBC in 4 Massachusetts communities	Mass screenings	Reminder postcards to see their physician	51.5% within 2–4 months	Reminder postcards yielded higher rate / Higher rates: old, higher BC, history of HBC, higher education
Maiman et al. (1992)	2,109 adults	Public screening	Referral by professional or lay communicator / Coupon offer, reminder letter, or control group (randomized)	No difference by communicator / 60.7% with coupon, / 57.7% with letter / 46.1% for controls	Interventions were effective *only* for "unaware" of HBC
Owen et al. (1990)	5,205 adults with HBC in Australia	Public screenings	Advice only (control) / Advice + follow-up booster letter and cookbook order form, after 4 weeks / Advice + follow-up + incentive (lottery ticket for prize) (randomized)	62.9% for advice / 59.1% for advice + FU / 61.4% for advice + FU + incentive	No significant differences between groups

Table 3.2. Behavior Change and Cholesterol Reduction

Citation	Sample	Design*	Diet Change?	Cholesterol Reduction?
Tymstra & Bieleman, 1987	107 Dutch men with HBC	One-time survey, NR	72% reported diet change due to screening & follow-up	Not reported
Kinlay & Heller, 1990	552 patients in Australian general medical practices	One-time survey, NR	46% with borderline BC 75% with HBC	Not reported
Rastam et al, 1988	424 adults with HBC	Pre-post, NR	66% reported "substantial dietary change"	Not reported
van Buerden et al, 1991 James et al., 1991	9,046 Australian adults	Pre-post, NR Follow-up n=2,183	80%, self-report	75% of follow-up group Mean change 8%
Hyman et al., 1991	188 adults in California with HBC and desirable BC levels	Pre-post, NR	Significant decreases in high chol., high sat fat foods, red meat, and cheese No significant diff. overall for HBC vs. desirable levels	3.2% mean decrease, no significant difference between levels

54

Havas et al., 1991	2,627 adults with HBC in Massachusetts	Follow-up survey of a random 15% R, C for follow-up reminders, but NR for counseling	Average 75% improvement in total dietary score	3.6% decrease with no MD 4.4% decrease with MD visit 8.8% decrease with medication
Gemson et al., 1990	232 employees with HBC levels	R, C High-frequency follow-up vs. low-frequency follow-up (HFF vs. LFF) (for n=137)	Greater change for HFF group; 24% improvement vs. 10% improvement	Average reduction of 8.3% No significant difference between groups
Ives et al., 1993	1197 Rural elderly	R, C with follow-up MD-treated vs. hospital-treated vs. control Follow-up n=75%	Not reported	Average 6% in all groups No significant effect of either intervention

*NR = nonrandomized; R, C = randomized, controlled trial

recommendations (diet and/or drugs), both because most investigations used relatively crude measures of dietary behavior and because
low-fat changes in eating patterns are reasonably well correlated with
BC-lowering effects (Glanz, 1985). Table 3.2 summarizes studies of
cholesterol screening and management that report on impact in terms
of dietary change and/or cholesterol reduction. Only two of the studies
reported experiments with different education/management strategies (Gemson, Sloan, Messeri, & Goldberg, 1990; Ives, Kuller, & Traven,
1993). Earlier reviews of cholesterol-education interventions in health
care settings, worksites, and communities during the 1980s also found
predominantly nonrandomized trials (Glanz, 1988; Wilson, 1991); most
of the randomized experiments with cholesterol change as the dependent variable were clinical trials of cholesterol-lowering therapy
(Glanz, 1988).

Virtually all of the studies found significant patient-reported levels
of dietary change. Likewise, all studies that included cholesterol measures (most of which were also patient-reported) found significant
reductions in BC. However, the two experimental investigations found
no difference in cholesterol reductions between treatment groups.
Although these results cannot be considered definitive indictments of
cholesterol screening and management programs, they underscore the
importance of using control groups. Perhaps the changes observed in
the nonrandomized studies reflect secular changes, the effect of an
attention placebo, or—most optimistically—the impact of simply going through the cholesterol screening and education process.

FUTURE DIRECTIONS IN RESEARCH AND PRACTICE

Since the mid-1980s, the available research on cholesterol screening
and management has grown rapidly. Because high blood cholesterol
is an important and highly prevalent risk factor, this area deserves
continuing attention. In the next few years, additional findings will
become available from studies under way, and they should expand
our understanding about cholesterol screening and its impact. There
are several important limitations of the research reviewed here. Many
studies lacked prescreening data and appropriate control or comparison groups, and thus observed outcomes could not necessarily be
attributed to the screening and/or feedback experience. Several studies
used poorly developed measures of psychological and cognitive factors and dietary behavior and relied solely on self-reports of cholesterol
levels. The form of feedback, advice, and follow-up that was used
varied widely across studies and could not be systematically com-

pared. Other common weaknesses included the use of self-selected volunteer participants, high dropout rates, and nonresponse or loss to follow-up after the test. Further, it is difficult to make direct comparisons among many of the studies because of different measures, designs, and data analyses.

There is a need for additional research that includes analyses of relevant subgroup characteristics, including gender, age, ethnicity, health care access, overweight status, and other cardiovascular risk factors. It would also be informative to further explore factors that moderate the impact of identification of both high and desirable-level cholesterol levels. Qualitative research may be useful in helping to reveal how people cope with a diagnosis of HBC, to increase our understanding of how to prevent or mitigate any decrements in psychological status and quality of life, and to help improve follow-up adherence and treatment compliance. Coordinated programs of research with multiple small-scale studies that combine investigations of short and long-term processes of coping and behavior change would be useful.

Future studies should try to design investigations to address, among others, these important evaluation questions:

1. Which elements of multi-component interventions, individually and in combination, are most effective in motivating patients to make changes in their behavior to reduce their cholesterol levels?
2. What is the relative impact of different strategies on various racial and ethnic groups, males and females, different age groups, and people of lower income and educational levels?
3. How do secular trends in cholesterol awareness and cholesterol levels interact with planned interventions?
4. What are the costs of false-positive screening results, in terms of worry and unnecessary use of health resources? What are the costs of false-negative results, in terms of delay in obtaining treatment and initiating therapeutic actions?

With respect to public health and health promotion practice, it is important to recognize that public screenings are widespread and to work to link them to medical care more effectively. More programs for low-income groups and minorities are warranted, as these groups are interested and express a positive attitude toward HBC control (Hyman, Simons-Morton, et al.,1993). Further, organizations that sponsor screening programs should be monitored for calibration of their instruments and for staff training and supervision. One policy question worthy of review concerns the use of ''borderline-high'' as a classification of BC levels—given the typical finding that follow-up rates in this category are lower than when people are informed that their levels are "high." Another important issue is what type of feedback should be provided at single-measure screenings. Further, the availability of reimbursement for both screening and outpatient treatment warrant review.

SUMMARY AND CONCLUSIONS

The studies that have been reviewed in this chapter suggest that psychological distress due to labeling individuals with high blood cholesterol is not a major problem. Recall of *general* results and advice is quite good among those who seek follow-up, though their memory of specific details such as the exact cholesterol level may be poor. (In this regard, the distinction between *necessary* information and other facts should be explored.) Follow-up among those identified as possibly having HBC at screenings is often inadequate, though higher risk levels predict better referral adherence. Another key factor that appears influential seems to be whether people had prior knowledge of elevated BC levels, though it is not clear how this knowledge influences subsequent thoughts and actions.

There is some evidence that cholesterol testing with simple dietary messages (and those disseminated through the mass media) may stimulate dietary changes. Trend data have shown that cholesterol levels in the United States are declining (Sempos et al., 1993; Johnson et al., 1993) and have also indicated increases in awareness and knowledge about cholesterol and cholesterol reduction since the inception of the National Cholesterol Education Program (NCEP) (Schucker et al., 1991; Frank, Winkleby et al., 1992). However, analyses of 171 studies of dietary assessments since 1920 indicate that total fat intake decreased from the mid-1960s to 1984 but has not continued to decrease since that time (Stephen & Wald, 1990). Consumption of some specific foods, such as low-fat milk and eggs, has changed in desirable directions, though (Thomas, 1991). Given the apparent secular trends, it is important to think how they can be built upon and accelerated in high-risk groups and individuals.

Currently, dietary guidelines for preventive health maintenance and for prevention of cardiovascular diseases and cancer stress common principles: limiting total fat consumption to 30% of calories or less, eating less saturated fat and cholesterol, consuming more foods that are high in dietary fiber, more fruits and vegetables, and avoiding overweight (American Heart Association, 1988; National Research

Council, 1989; USDHHS, 1988; USDA/USDHHS, 1990; USDHHS, 1991). Inclusion of preventive nutrition counseling, as well as risk factor testing, within routine medical care will require gradual, systematic efforts of multiple sectors (US Preventive Services Task Force, 1989; Thomas, 1991; Remington, 1990).

The application of findings from research reviewed here is neither clear nor unidirectional. A diagnosis of high blood cholesterol does not appear to cause major psychological repercussions for most people. This may be due to its being highly prevalent and thus virtually commonplace. Although heart disease is the leading cause of death in industrialized nations, it does not evoke as much fear as cancer and HIV/AIDS. The major therapy, dietary change, is burdensome and difficult for some but seldom causes untoward side effects.

Major challenges lie ahead in the development of both practical, accurate, and reliable screening and follow-up programs. Further research should be the basis for better understanding the psychosocial impact of cholesterol screening and management. Strategies to promote long-term risk factor reduction, better quality of life, reduced morbidity, and premature mortality are potential benefits of this line of inquiry.

REFERENCES

Allen, S., Bache-Wiig, M., & Hunninghake D. (1992). Patient perceptions about the influence of cholesterol on heart disease. *American Journal of Preventive Medicine, 8*, 30–36.

American Heart Association. (1988). Dietary guidelines for healthy American adults. *Circulation, 77*, 721A–724A.

Axelson M., & Brinberg D. (1992). The measurement and conceptualization of nutrition knowledge. *J Nutr Educ* 24, 239–246.

Boyle, K., Lenhert, E., Porter, L., & Pryor, B. (1992). Measuring up: Quality assurance for cholesterol screening programs in Ohio. *American Journal Public Heath, 82*, 1687–1688.

Brett, A. (1991). Psychologic effects of the diagnosis and treatment of hypercholesterolemia: Lessons from case studies. *American Journal of Medicine, 91*, 642–647.

Burke, J., & Fischer, P. (1988). A clinician's guide to the office measurement of cholesterol. *JAMA, 259*, 3444–3448.

Burns, R., Stoy, D., Feied, C., Nash, E., Smith, M. (1991) Cholesterol screening in the emergency department. *Journal of General Internal Medicine, 6*, 210–215.

Centers for Disease Control. (1992). Cholesterol screening and awareness—Behavioral risk factor surveillance system, 1990. *MMWR, 41*, 669, 675–678.

———. (1990). Factors related to cholesterol screening, cholesterol level awareness—United States, 1989. *MMWR, 39*, 633–637.

Consensus Conference. (1985). Lowering blood cholesterol to prevent heart disease. *JAMA, 253*, 2080–2086.

Cooper, G., Myers, G., Smith, S., & Schlant, R. (1992). Blood lipid measurements: Variations and practical utility. *JAMA, 267*, 1642–1660.

Croyle, R., Sun, Y., & Louie, D. (1993). Psychological minimization of cholesterol test results: Moderators of appraisal in college students and community residents. *Health Psychology, 12*, 503–507.

Ernst, N. D., & Cleeman, J. (1988). Reducing high blood cholesterol levels: Recommendations from the National Cholesterol Education Program. *J Nutr Educ 20*, 23–29.

Expert Panel on Detection, Evaluation, and Treatment of High Blood Cholesterol in Adults. (1993). Summary of the Second Report of the National Cholesterol Education Program (NCEP) Expert Panel on Detection, Evaluation, and Treatment of High Blood Cholesterol in Adults (Adult Treatment Panel II). *JAMA, 269*, 3015–3023.

Fischer, P., Guinan, K., Burke, J., Karp, W., & Richards, J. (1990). Impact of a public cholesterol screening program. *Archives of Internal Medicine, 150*, 2567–2572.

Fitzgerald, S., Gibbens, S., & Agnew, J. (1991). Evaluation of referral completion after a workplace screening program. *American Journal of Preventive Medicine, 7*, 335–340.

Food Marketing Institute. (1992). *Trends: Consumer Attitudes and the Supermarket.* Washington, DC: Food Marketing Institute.

Frank, E., Winkleby, M., Fortmann, S., Rockhill, B., & Farquhar, J. (1992). Improved cholesterol-related knowledge and behavior and plasma cholesterol levels in adults during the 1980s. *JAMA, 268*, 1566–1572.

Frank, E., Winkleby, M., Fortmann, S., & Farquhar, J. (1993). Cardiovascular disease risk factors: Improvements in knowledge and behavior in the 1980s. *American Journal of Public Health, 83*, 590–593.

Gans, K., Lasater, T., Linnan, L., LaPane, K., & Carleton, R. (1990). A cholesterol screening and education program: Differences between older and younger adults. *J Nutr Educ 22*, 275–283.

Gans, K., Lefebvre, R., Lasater, T., Nelson, D., Loberti, P., & Carleton, R. (1989). Measuring blood cholesterol in the community: Participant characteristics by site. *Health Educ Res 4*, 399–406.

Gemson, D., Sloan, R., Messeri, P., & Goldberg, I. (1990). A public health model for cardiovascular risk reduction. *Archives of Internal Medicine, 150*, 985–989.

Giles, W., Anda, R., Jones, D., Serdula, M., Merritt, R., & DeStefano, F. (1993). Recent trends in the identification and treatment of high blood cholesterol by physicians. *JAMA, 269*, 1133–1138.

Glanz, K. (1985). Nutrition education for risk factor reduction and patient education: A review. *Preventive Medicine, 14*, 721–752.

———. (1988). Patient and public education for cholesterol reduction: A review of strategies and issues. *Patient Education and Counseling, 12*, 235–257.

———. (1990). The cholesterol controversy and health education: A response to the critics. *Patient Education and Counseling, 1990; 16*, 89–95.

Glanz, K., Brekke, M., Hoffman, E., Admire, J., McComas, K., & Mullis, R. (1990). Patient reactions to nutrition education for cholesterol reduction. *American Journal of Preventive Medicine, 6*, 311–317.

Glanz, K., & Gilboy, M. B. (1992). Physicians, preventive care, and applied nutrition: Selected literature. *Academic Medicine, 67*, 776–781.

Glanz, K., & Scholl, T. (1982). Intervention strategies to improve adherence among hypertensives: Review and recommendations. *Pat Couns Health Educ 4,* 14–28.

Gordon, R., Klag, M., & Whelton, P. (1990). Community cholesterol screening: Impact of labeling on participant behavior. *Archives of Internal Medicine, 150,* 1957–1960.

Gotto, A., et al. (1990). The cholesterol facts: A summary of the evidence relating dietary fats, serum cholesterol, and coronary heart disease. *Circulation, 81,* 1721–1733.

Grover S., Abrahamowicz, M., Joseph, L., Brewer, C., Coupal, L., & Suissa, S. (1992). The benefits of treating hyperlipidemia to prevent coronary heart disease: Estimating changes in life expectancy and morbidity. *JAMA, 267,* 816–822.

Gwynne, J. (1991). Measuring and knowing: The trouble with cholesterol and decision making. *JAMA, 266,* 1696–1698.

Harlan, W. R., & Stross, J. K. (1985). An educational view of a national initiative to lower plasma lipid levels. *JAMA, 235,* 2087–2090.

Havas, S., Bishop, R., Koumjian, L., Reisman, J., & Wozenski, S. (1992). Performance of the Reflotron in Massachusetts' Model Systems for Blood Cholesterol Screening Program. *American Journal of Public Health, 82,* 458–461.

Havas, S., Greenland, P., Wones, R., & Schucker, B. (1989). Addressing unanswered questions about population cholesterol screenings: The Model Systems for Blood Cholesterol Screening Program. *American Journal of Preventive Medicine, 5,* 337–346.

Havas, S., Koumjian, L., Reisman, J., Hsu, L., & Wozenski, S. (1991). Results of the Massachusetts Model Systems for Blood Cholesterol Screening Project. *JAMA, 266,* 375–381.

Havas, S., Reisman, J., Hsu, L., & Koumjian, L. (1991). Does cholesterol screening result in negative labeling effects? Results of the Massachusetts Model Systems for Blood Cholesterol Screening Project. *Archives of Internal Medicine, 151,* 113–119.

Hulley, S., & Newman, T. (1992). Position statement: Cholesterol screening in children is not indicated, even with positive family history. *Journal of the American College of Nutrition, 11,* 20S–22S.

Hyman, D., Flora, J., Reynolds, K., Johannson, M., & Farquhar, J. (1991). The impact of public cholesterol screening on diet, general well-being, and physician referral. *American Journal of Preventive Medicine, 7,* 268–272.

Hyman, D., Paradis, G., & Flora, J. (1992). A comparison of participants and nonparticipants in a worksite cholesterol screening. *American Journal of Health Promotion, 7,* 137–141.

Hyman, D., Simons-Morton, D., Ho, K., Dunn, J., & Rubovits, D. (1993). Cholesterol-related knowledge, attitudes and behaviors in a low-income, urban population. *American Journal of Preventive Medicine, 9,* 282–289.

Ives, D., Kuller, L., & Traven, N. (1993). Use and outcomes of a cholesterol-lowering intervention for rural elderly subjects. *American Journal of Preventive Medicine, 9,* 274–281.

Jacobs, D. R., & Blackburn, H. (1993). Models of effects of low blood cholesterol on the public health: Implications for practice and policy. *Circulation, 87,* 1033–1036.

James, R., van Beurden, E., Tyler, C., Henrikson, D., & Ash, S. (1991). Blood cholesterol reduction following community-based screening and dietary counseling. *J Nutr Educ 23,* 104–109.

Johnson, C., Rifkind, B., Sempos, T., et al. (1993). Declining serum total cholesterol levels among US adults: The National Health and Nutrition Examination Surveys. *JAMA, 269,* 3002–3008.

Kinlay, S. (1988). High cholesterol levels: Is mass screening the best option? *Medical Journal of Australia, 148,* 635–637.

Kinlay, S., & Heller, R. (1990). Effectiveness and hazards of case finding for a high cholesterol concentration. *British Medical Journal, 300,* 1545–1547.

Koch, D., Hassemer, D., Wiebe, D., & Laessig, R. (1988). Testing cholesterol accuracy: Performance of several common laboratory instruments. *JAMA, 260,* 2552–2557.

Lasater, T., Lefebvre, R., Assaf, A., Saritelli, A., & Carleton, R. (1987). Rapid measurement of blood cholesterol: Evaluation of a new instrument. *American Journal of Preventive Medicine, 3,* 311–316.

Lefebvre, R., Hursey, K., & Carleton, R. (1988). Labeling of participants in high blood pressure screening programs: Implications for blood cholesterol screenings. *Archives of Internal Medicine, 148,* 1993–1997.

Lefebvre, R., Linnan, L., Sundaram, S., & Ronan, A. (1990). Counseling strategies for blood cholesterol screening programs: Recommendations for practice. *Patient Education and Counseling, 16,* 97–108.

Lerman, C., Trock, B., Rimer, B., Jepson, C., Boyce, A., & Engstrom, P. (1991). Psychological and behavioral implications of abnormal mammograms. *Annals of Internal Medicine, 114,* 657–661.

Levy, A., Fein, S., & Stephenson, M. (1993). Nutrition knowledge levels about dietary fats and cholesterol: 1983–1988. *J Nutr Educ 25,* 60–66.

Ley, P. (1987). Cognitive variables and noncompliance. *Journal Compliance Health Care, 1,* 171–188.

MacDonald, L., Sackett, D., Haynes, R., & Taylor, D. (1984). Labelling in hypertension: A review of the behavioral and psychological consequences. *J Chron Dis 37,* 933–942.

Maiman, L., Greenland, P., Hildreth, N., & Cox, C. (1991). Patterns of physicians' treatment for referral patients from public cholesterol screening. *American Journal of Preventive Medicine, 7,* 273–279.

———. (1992). Improving referral compliance after public cholesterol screening. *American Journal of Public Health, 82,* 804–809.

Muldoon, M., & Manuck, S. (1992). Health through cholesterol reduction: Are there unforeseen risks? *Ann Behav Med 14,* 101–108.

Naughton, M., Luepker, R., & Strickland, D. (1990). The accuracy of portable cholesterol analyzers in public screening programs. *JAMA, 263,* 1213–1217.

National Cholesterol Education Program. (1990). Report of the expert panel on population strategies for blood cholesterol reduction. Bethesda, MD: National Institutes of Health (NIH Publ. No. 90-3046).

National Research Council. (1989). *Diet and Health: Implications for Reducing Chronic Disease Risk.* Washington, DC: National Academy Press.

NCEP Coordinating Committee, National Cholesterol Education program. (1987). *Public Screening for Measuring Blood Cholesterol—Issues for Special Concern.* Bethesda, MD: NHLBI Information Center.

Owen, N., James, R., Henrikson, D., van Beurden, E. (1990). Community cholesterol screenings: The impact of follow-up letters and incentives on retest rates and biometric changes in follow-up screenings. *American Journal of Health Promotion, 5,* 58–62.

Pearson, T., Bowlin, S., & Sigmund, W. (1990). Screening for hypercholesterolemia. *Annual Review of Medicine, 41,* 177–186.

Polednak, A. (1992). Awareness and use of blood cholesterol tests in 40–74-year-olds by educational level. *Public Health Reports, 107,* 345–351.

Rastam, L., Frick, J., & Gullberg, B. (1991). Work absenteeism in men who are labelled hypercholesterolaemic at screening. *European Heart Journal, 12,* 1316–1320.

Rastam, L., Luepker, R., & Pirie, P. (1988). Effect of screening and referral on follow-up and treatment of high blood cholesterol levels. *American Journal of Preventive Medicine, 4,* 244–248.

Remington, R. D. (1990). From preventive policy to preventive practice. *Preventive Medicine, 19,* 105–113.

Report of the National Cholesterol Education Program Expert Panel on Detection, Evaluation, and Treatment of High Blood Cholesterol in Adults. (1988). *Archives of Internal Medicine, 148,* 36–69.

Schucker, B., Bailey, K., Heimbach, J. T., et al. (1987). Change in public perspective on cholesterol and heart disease: Results from national physician and public surveys. *MAMA, 258,* 3527–3531.

Schucker, B., Wittes, J. T., Santanello, N. C., et al. (1991). Change in cholesterol awareness and action: Results from national physician and public surveys. *Archives of Internal Medicine, 151,* 666–673.

Sempos, C. T., Cleeman, J. I., Carroll, M. D., et al. (1993). Prevalence of high blood cholesterol among US adults: An update based on guidelines from the Second Report of the National Cholesterol Education Program Adult Treatment Panel. *JAMA, 269,* 3009–3014.

Sprafka, J. M., Burke, G. L., Folson, A. R., & Hahn, L. P. (1989). Hypercholesterolemia prevalence, awareness, and treatment in blacks and whites. *Preventive Medicine, 18,* 423–432.

Stave, G., Winslow, B., & Conner, G. (1991). Variability in cholesterol measurements in a worksite cholesterol screening program. *American Journal of Preventive Medicine, 7,* 406–409.

Stephen, A. M., & Wald, N. J. (1990). Trends in individual consumption of dietary fat in the United States. *American Journal of Clinical Nutrition, 52,* 457–469.

Thomas, P. (Ed.). (1991). *Improving America's Diet and Health: From Recommendations to Action.* Washington, DC: National Academy Press.

Tymstra, R., & Bieleman, B. (1987). The psychosocial impact of mass screening for cardiovascular risk factors. *Family Practice, 4,* 287–290.

US Department of Agriculture and US Department of Health and Human Services. (1990). *Nutrition and Your Health: Dietary Guidelines for Americans (3rd ed.).* Washington, DC: US Govt. Printing Office.

US Department of Health and Human Services. (1987). *Current Status of Cholesterol Measurement in Clinical Laboratories in the United States: A Statement from the National Cholesterol Education Program.* Bethesda, Md.: National Heart, Lung, and Blood Institute.

———. (1991). *Healthy People 2000: National Health Promotion and Disease Prevention Objectives.* Washington, DC: US Govt. Printing Office (DHHS Publ. No. PHS 91-50213).

———. (1990). *Recommendations for Improving Cholesterol Measurement: A Report*

From the Laboratory Standardization Panel of the National Cholesterol Education Program. Bethesda, Md.: National Heart, Lung, and Blood Institute (NIH Publ. No. PHS 90-2964).

————. (1988). *The Surgeon General's Report on Nutrition and Health*. Washington, DC: US Govt. Printing Office (DHHS Publ. No. PHS-88-50210).

US Preventive Services Task Force. (1989). *Guide to Clinical Preventive Services*. Baltimore, Md: Williams & Wilkins.

van Beurden, E., James, R., Henrikson, D., & Tyler, C. (1991). Implementing a large scale community-based health promotion campaign with a limited budget. *Health Promotion Journal of Australia, 1*, 35–39.

Wilson, M. (1991). Cholesterol reduction in workplace and community settings. *Journal of Community Health, 16*, 49–65.

Wilson, M., & Edmunson, J. (1991). Prevalence of hypercholesterolemia in a national worksite sample. *American Journal of Preventive Medicine, 7*, 280–284.

4

Psychosocial Impact of Cancer Screening

CARYN LERMAN
BARBARA K. RIMER

Basic and medical science investigations have identified a growing number of factors that predispose to cancer. Risks related to precancerous lesions (Hutchinson et al., 1980) and to occupational exposures (Mason, Prorok, Neeld, & Vogler, 1986) have been researched widely. A variety of population-based and worksite screening programs have been implemented to identify individuals at increased risk for cancer by virtue of these factors. However, such programs are not without psychological costs (Lerman, Rimer, & Engstrom, 1991). The potential psychological sequelae of cancer screening are of particular concern, as these effects can deter adherence to recommended regimens for continued surveillance (Lerman, Rimer, Trock, Balshem, & Engstrom, 1990; Kash, Holland, Halper, & Miller, 1992; Lerman et al., 1993). Despite this, there has been little attention to the psychosocial impact of cancer screening.

Here, we review the literature on the psychological and behavioral impact of programs for early cancer detection and notification of carcinogenic occupational exposures. Articles were identified through a search of the MEDLINE bibliographic database, as well as searches of reference lists in published articles. Implications of these findings for improving adherence and reducing cancer morbidity and mortality will be emphasized. Suggestions for patient education and future research directions also will be discussed.

CANCER SCREENING: THE IMPACT OF ABNORMAL RESULTS

Early detection and treatment of asymptomatic neoplasms and precursor lesions can reduce cancer morbidity and mortality (Guzick, 1978; Tabar & Dean, 1987; Dales, Friedman, & Colleen, 1979). On the basis of these and other epidemiological data, the National Cancer Institute has established a nationwide goal to reduce cancer mortality by 50% by the year 2000 (Greenwald & Sondik, 1986). Major efforts have been directed toward screening objectives that emphasize regular mammography and Papanicolaou (Pap) tests. With improvements in patient and provider education, rates of adherence to these early detection regimens are increasing (Lerman, Rimer, & Engstrom, 1989). As a consequence of more widespread use, however, the incidence of positive test results will rise. For example, the proportion of inconclusive or abnormal mammograms in large-scale breast screening programs is as high as 20% (Winchester, Lasky, Sylvester, & Mayer, 1988; Lerman, Trock, et al., 1991). Thus, if 38% of the 48 million American women aged 40 years and over have a mammogram (Dawson & Thompson, 1990), the estimated number of indeterminant or positive examinations would be over 3 million.

While breast cancer screening has the potential to reduce morbidity and mortality, there may be significant negative psychological sequelae of this experience. One study examined participants of a breast-screening program offered through a health maintenance organization (HMO) (Lerman, Trock, et al., 1991). The sample included women with normal mammograms (n = 121), low-suspicion abnormal mammograms (n = 119), and high suspicion abnormal mammograms (n = 68), but not women with breast cancer. Psychological responses to screening were assessed by telephone interview 3 months after receipt of mammogram results. Women with high-suspicion mammograms had substantial mammography-related anxiety (47%) and worries about breast cancer (41%). Such worries affected the moods (26%) and daily functioning (17%) of these women, despite diagnostic evaluation excluding malignancy. For each psychological variable, a consistent significant increase in psychological distress was observed with degree of mammogram abnormality.

Two other studies revealed similar effects of abnormal mammograms. Ellman and colleagues (1989) used the General Health Questionnaire to assess psychiatric morbidity in 302 women who received routine mammography, 300 women who had received false-positive mammogram results, and 150 women who were symptomatic for benign breast disease. Women with false-positive mammography results and those with symptomatic benign conditions exhibited significantly higher levels of anxiety than women with normal results. Overall, psychiatric morbidity was documented in 25% of women with normal results, 30% of women with false-positive results, and 35% of women with symptomatic benign conditions. After 3 months, levels of morbidity had returned to baseline among women with false-positive results, but persisted in the symptomatic benign group.

As part of a mass mammography screening program in Sweden, Gram, Lund, and Slenker (1990) evaluated 160 women with false-positive mammogram results and a random sample of 250 women with negative results. Six months following screening, these women completed self-report questionnaires of their psychological responses to the screening process. Additional in-person interviews were conducted 1 year later. Compared with 209 women with negative screening results, a substantial proportion of women with false-positive results reported moderate anxiety (40% vs. 22%) 6 months after the test. Anxiety levels decreased in both groups after 18 months (29% vs. 13%), and there were no long-term effects on sleep patterns or general well-being. In addition, the false-positive group reported a statistically significant decrease in their quality of life during the diagnostic workup period. Overall, however, most women regarded the false-positive mammogram as one of many minor life stressors. A substantial proportion also noted that the experience had an overall positive impact on their lives.

Two other studies using standardized psychological measures found no evidence for psychological differences between women with breast problems and women in the general population (Romsaas, Malec, Jarenkoski, Trump, & Wolberg, 1986; Morris & Greer, 1982). Romsaas and colleagues studied a diverse group of clinic patients who were seeking diagnosis regarding breast problems. From an original group of 412 women, 322 valid questionnaire forms were received. These included measures of breast cancer knowledge, along with the Profile of Mood Status (POMS) and Health Locus Control Scale (HLCS). Women whose diagnosis of breast cancer was known scored higher on several POMS subscales, including tension-anxiety, depression-dejection, anger-hostility, confusion-bewilderment, and total mood disturbance. Patients with unknown diagnoses scored higher on vigor-activity. Overall, diagnosis-known patients showed more distress than diagnosis-unknown patients. The authors cautioned that the apparent lack of distress among the diagnosis-unknown group might reflect the older age and self-referral biases.

Morris and Greer (1982) also studied patients at a breast clinic and administered several personality tests, including the Eysenck Personality Questionnaire (ESPQ) and the Spielberger State-Trait Anxiety Inventory (STAI). Of 1,010 patients receiving questionnaires, 834 returned them. The results showed that these patients did not have elevated levels of anxiety. It may be that women who self-refer to breast clinics are more likely to employ active and adaptive coping mechanisms in the face of ambiguity. Similarly, these women also are more likely to be white and well-educated and to have higher incomes. Thus, they are the very group who reflect higher profiles of compliance on most cancer control behaviors (Lerman et al., 1989).

The psychological effects of receiving positive Pap test results were evaluated in a study of women attending an inner-city medical clinic. One hundred and six women with normal Pap results were compared with 118 women who were referred for colposcopic examination for follow-up of positive test results (Lerman, Miller, et al., 1991). All patients were interviewed by telephone 3 months after they had received their test results. Women with positive results showed statistically significant elevations in worries about cancer, as well as impairments in mood, daily activities, sexual interest, and sleep patterns. For example, about 45% of women with positive results reported that they worried about developing cervical cancer and 13% of women had impairments in their daily activities due to these worries. These psychological effects were more pronounced among women who did not adhere to the recommended colposcopy examination. These women did not avail themselves of the opportunity to learn that abnormal cervical lesions can be treated easily and that cervical cancer can be prevented. It is not surprising that in the absence of such information, uncertainty about diagnosis and cancer anxiety remained high.

Similar findings were obtained in a descriptive study of the cervical cancer screening process. McDonald, Neutens, Fischer, and Jessee (1989) followed 20 women from the time of receipt of positive Pap test results through diagnosis and treatment. Patients completed self-report questionnaires on four consecutive visits to the colposcopy clinic. Prior to colposcopy examination, the predominant concern was fear of cancer (100% of women). Cancer concerns diminished only slightly across visits (59% by the fourth visit). After surgery, loss of sexual function was rated as a primary concern by at least one half of patients at all four visits.

While these studies indicate that cervical cancer screening can produce significant psychological consequences, a study of Reelick, De Haes, and Schuurman (1984) suggests that such effects may not be long lasting. As part of a mass cervical cancer screening program in Norway, they evaluated the psychological responses of 175 women with positive Pap smear results. Compared with women who had negative results, these women exhibited significant mood disturbance within the few days following receipt of results. Psychological distress persisted after definitive treatment in 35% of women. However, there were no significant effects of a positive result observed at 6-month follow-up. Again, it may be that the uncertainty about cancer is minimized with time and receipt of information about cervical cancer prevention.

Due to controversy over the benefits of early detection for ovarian cancer, little attention has been directed to the psychosocial impact of screening for this disease. However, one recent study examined the psychological responses of women with a family history of ovarian cancer who self-referred to an ovarian cancer screening program in the United Kingdom (Wardle et al., 1993). Subjects completed assessments of information-seeking coping style (Miller Behavioral Style Scale, Miller, & Mangan, 1983) prior to screening and assessments of depression, anxiety, and general well-being at prescreening and at a 3-month follow-up. Psychological distress was reduced significantly for women who received negative results. Among women with positive results, elevations in distress were observed only for those with information-seeking coping styles. The importance of individual differences in coping styles is also supported by a recent study of attitudes and expectations about genetic testing for cancer among women at high risk for ovarian cancer (Lerman, Daly, Masney, & Balshem, 1994). In this study, women with information-seeking coping styles were significantly more likely to anticipate adverse psychological consequences of genetic testing than other high-risk women.

IMPACT OF PSYCHOLOGICAL DISTRESS ON CANCER SCREENING BEHAVIORS

The potential of cancer screening to produce short-term psychological sequelae is of particular concern because of the possible impact of psychological distress on subsequent health behavior. Although the perception that one is "at risk" can lead to enhanced vigilance and protective behavior to reduce a health threat (Nerenz & Leventhal, 1983), extreme levels of distress actually can interfere with adherence behavior (Janis & Feshbach, 1953). For example, anxiety and cancer worries have been associated with lower rates of mammography (Lerman et al., 1990; Lerman et al., 1993) as well as reductions in breast self-examination (BSE) frequency (Alagna, Morokoff, Bevett, & Reddy, 1987) and clinical breast examination (CBE) (Kash et al., 1992). One of these studies (Alagna et al., 1987) examined 32 women at high risk for breast cancer on the basis of family history and 61 women at low risk. Measures were obtained for breast self-examination (BSE) practice and a variety of attitudinal items related to breast cancer (e.g., severity). Although high-risk women were more knowledgeable about breast cancer, they were less likely to practice monthly BSE. Because the high-risk group was more anxious about breast cancer, they may have avoided BSE because they feared finding something.

Two of these studies focused on the breast cancer screening practices of women at high risk for this disease. Kash et al. (1992) examined psychological distress and adherence among 217 women with a family history of breast cancer. Health Belief Model variables and measures derived from Fear Arousing Communications Theory were used along with a number of standard psychological measures (e.g., Impact of Event Scale [IES] and Brief Symptom Inventory [BSI]). On the BSI, 27% of the women had levels of psychological distress consistent with a need for counseling. Women who had more barriers to adherence and fewer social supports had significantly more distress. Those with more anxiety were significantly less likely to get CBEs. Likewise, as the frequency of anxiety increased, BSE practice decreased. In a similar sample, Lerman et al. (1993) showed that serious breast cancer worries were associated with lower rates of adherence to age-specific mammography screening guidelines. This effect was especially pronounced for women with less formal education.

The studies by Alagna et al. (1987), Kash et al. (1992), and Lerman et al. (1993) suggest that women defined as high risk on the basis of their family history may be an important screening subgroup with greater anxiety and distress. The diagnosis of cancer in a close relative tends to produce substantial psychological distress in most women (Kelly, 1991). Moreover, a substantial proportion of persons with a family history of cancer are misinformed about their personal risk status and do not adhere to recommended cancer screening following the relative's diagnosis (Houts, Wojtkowiak, Simmonds, Weinberg, & Heitjan, 1991). These women may require more intensive interventions to educate them about their personal risk and to minimize their anxiety about cancer screening (Lerman, Rimer, & Engstrom, 1991). These efforts may be especially beneficial for women with less formal education (Lerman et al., 1993).

Two recent studies examined breast screening practices among women at risk due to prior abnormal mammogram results. Lerman and colleagues studied 308 women aged 50 and older approximately 3 months following a screening mammogram. Psychological responses and frequency of breast self-examination were evaluated by telephone interview. The results showed a curvilinear relationship between breast cancer worries and BSE practice among women with abnormal mammograms (Lerman, Trock, Rimer, Jepson, et al., 1991). Specifically, women with moderate levels of breast cancer worries were more likely to practice monthly BSE than women with either high or low levels of worry. These findings suggest that intermediate levels of worry may be optimal for motivating continued BSE practice.

Lerman and colleagues followed these subjects prospectively for 1 year to examine prospective mammography adherence. The results showed that the majority of women (77%) who had initial abnormal mammograms did receive a screening mammogram the following year (Lerman, Trock, Rimer, Boyce, et al. 1991). Contrary to predictions, breast cancer worries following the initial mammogram were not associated with a reduced likelihood of subsequent screening. In fact, women who were no longer concerned about their previous abnormal mammogram results were the *least likely* to obtain subsequent mammograms. Thus, some degree of concern or anxiety about breast cancer might heighten women's vigilance and motivate them to seek reassurance through repetitive breast screening.

Another study suggests that the impact of abnormal breast screening results on subsequent adherence may be influenced by prior patterns of screening behavior. Haefner, Becker, Janz, and Rutt (1989) evaluated the impact of a negative breast biopsy on subsequent BSE practice among 655 women. Women who had practiced BSE regularly prior to detection of the lump were compared with those who had not practiced regularly. Previously regular BSE practicers were significantly more likely to reduce their frequency of BSE practice following the negative biopsy than controls (women attending a general medical clinic). In contrast, women who had not been regular BSE practicers were signficantly more likely to increase their frequency of BSE practice. As the authors noted, these different groups of women may have received different messages from health care professionals during the process of resolving their diagnoses.

Other studies suggest that psychological distress following cervical cancer screening can deter adherence to diagnostic follow-up among women with positive Pap test results. For example, in the cervical screening study described above (Lerman, Miller, et al., 1991), women who adhered to diagnostic follow-up (colposcopy examination) did not exhibit heightened worry or impairment, whereas those who did not adhere reported persistent psychological distress. Additionally, in a study of 90 women referred for colposcopic examination, psychological barriers to adherence were reported by 35% of women. Twenty-four percent of women who did not adhere to colposcopy cited fear of cancer as the primary barrier and 11% were deterred by anxiety about the procedure itself (Lerman et al., 1992).

This research suggests that the relationship between anxiety and cancer screening behaviors is rather complex. Some studies have shown that anxiety can deter adherence (Kash et al., 1992; Lerman et al., 1993); others suggest that moderate levels of concern can facilitate subsequent screening behaviors (Lerman, Trock, Rimer, Boyce, et al., 1991). This inconsistency may be due to differences in study populations. For example, Kash et al. (1992) studied women who had self-referred to a breast prevention clinic due to concerns about their personal risk of breast cancer. Such women are likely to experience anxiety and cancer concerns that are elevated relative to women in the general population.

The Self-Regulation Model of Health Behavior (Leventhal, 1965) provides a useful framework for addressing this complex issue. This model suggests that moderate levels of perceived health threat (e.g., abnormal test result or diagnosis of cancer in a relative) will motivate persons to adopt a health practice in order to reduce anxiety that is generated by the health threat. Other work suggests that persons with minimal levels of anxiety may hold "optimistic biases" regarding personal risk and, as such, will be less likely to adopt preventive health practices (Weinstein, 1989). Thus, although excessive cancer-related anxiety might deter adoption of cancer screening practices, at least minimal levels of anxiety might be necessary to motivate these behaviors. In order to maximize the effectiveness of interventions to promote continued adherence to cancer screening, it will be important to determine what level of threat in health communication is optimal for motivating adherence while minimizing psychological distress.

INTERVENTIONS FOR PERSONS WITH ABNORMAL CANCER SCREENING RESULTS

The research reviewed above suggests that proper education and counseling of persons with positive results is essential to prevent excessive psychological distress and to promote continued adherence. Psycho-educational interventions for these populations have been tested in only a few studies. For example, a recent randomized trial was conducted to evaluate the impact of mailed psychoeducational materials on adherence to subsequent annual mammography among women with abnormal mammograms. The intervention was a 12-page booklet that described the meaning of abnormal mammograms and the necessity of continued screening. Suggestions for managing mammography-related anxiety also were included. The results showed a 13% increment in subsequent mammography adherence among women who received this intervention. This effect was independent of all sociodemographic and medical confounder variables examined (Lerman, et al., 1992).

Similar effects of written materials have been documented for women with positive Pap test results (Wilkenson, Jones, & McBride, 1990; Paskett, White, Carter, & Chu, 1990). Wilkenson et al. (1990) compared a standard computerized letter notifying patients of an abnormal Pap test result (n = 31 patients) compared to a leaflet and more personalized letter (n = 29 patients). The women who received the standard letter were significantly more likely to believe they had cancer and to believe their health had deteriorated. These patients also had higher mean scores on State-Trait Anxiety Inventory (STAI). Paskett et al. (1990) showed that a carefully developed brochure resulted in significantly higher compliance with follow-up among women with abnormal Pap tests who required further workups. This written communication highlighted specific areas of patient concerns that may function as barriers to adherence, including cancer fears and aversion to medical procedures.

More intensive intervention efforts may be necessary for those women with abnormal results who remain recalcitrant to follow-up. For example, a recent study tested a brief telephone barriers counseling intervention for women with abnormal Pap tests who did not adhere to their initial colposcopy appointment. Standardized prompts were used to elicit barriers to adherence, and scripted health education responses were delivered. Women who were anxious about the procedure were given suggestions to manage anxiety, and practical suggestions were given to women who reported transportation or financial barriers. This intervention produced a 24% increment in adherence to subsequent colposcopy compared with standard care (Lerman et al., 1992).

IMPACT OF OCCUPATIONAL EXPOSURES

Growing numbers of substances in the environment and workplace are being implicated in carcinogenesis. For example, it is estimated that about 2.5 million workers have had some exposure to asbestos, a silicate fiber linked to carcinomas of the lung and colon and to mesothelioma (United States Department of Health and Human Services [USDHHS], 1989). Benzidine and beta-naphthylamine (BNA), used widely in the chemical and dye industries, also are recognized bladder carcinogens (Mason et al., 1986). About 2,000 workers may have been exposed to benzidine directly, and 79,000 have been exposed to benzidine-based dyes (USDHHS, 1989). In addition, workers involved in pattern making for mass-produced items have a twofold to threefold increased risk of colon cancer (Hoar et al., 1986). Finally, there is evidence that lifestyle factors, such as cigarette smoking and alcohol intake, act synergistically with such toxins in the development of malignancies (Flanders & Rothman, 1982). Thus, the recommendations for exposed persons may include advice to obtain screening procedures and appropriate follow-up as well as to change behaviors that exacerbate the risk of disease.

Increasingly, workers are being notified and screened for potential exposures to these and other substances. However, there has been a great deal of controversy over procedures and consequences of such programs (Schulte & Ringen, 1984). Notification and screening of workers at risk has the potential to increase the likelihood that they will participate in programs for early detection and will adopt recommended preventive practices such as protective clothing and smoking cessation. However, some have argued that the potential psychological costs of these programs might outweigh these benefits (Bayer, 1986; Coon & Polakoff, 1982).

Several studies have examined the possible psychosocial impact of worker cancer risk notification and screening for cancer risk. Denial and minimization of risk were the predominant psychological reactions of workers with asbestos-related mesothelioma (Lebovitz, Chahinian, Gorzynski, & Holland, 1981). Therefore, it is not surprising that notification did not lead to adoption of preventive health practices. None of the smokers quit smoking (80% of sample were smokers), and no worker reported that screening prompted him or her to visit a physician. A second study using a psychiatric symptom rating scale to assess the impact of notification documented relatively high levels of distress among workers exposed to vinyl chloride (Sands, Newby, & Greenberg, 1981). However, the results of these studies must be interpreted cautiously because the populations studied had stressors other than notification. For example, workers in both studies had already been informed of suspicious findings or of a malignancy. Thus, it is not possible to isolate the impact of notification from the impact of diagnosis.

Other research in this area does not support the adverse effects of worker notification and screening programs. For example, Meyerowitz, Sullivan, and Premeau (1989) found only mild distress in workers who were informed of asbestos exposure and given an opportunity for medical screening. Hornsby and colleagues (1985) studied the psychological impact of notifying workers exposed to BNA. Scores on measures of stress symptoms and psychopathology, administered within 4 weeks of notification, were not elevated relative to normative samples. However, one limitation of these studies is the lack of a control group. Another study comparing the responses of workers notified of asbestos risks with those of a nonnotified control group did not show any significant differences in emotional responses or in health practices (Houts & McDougall, 1988).

Taken together, studies on the consequences of notifying and screening workers exposed to carcinogens do not provide evidence for significant adverse emotional reactions. In fact, minimization and denial of risks among workers appear to be the predominant reactions. This may be due to the fact that one's livelihood could be dependent upon continued exposure. Unfortunately, however, such coping strategies can contribute to avoidance of screening (Meyerowitz et al., 1989) and can interfere with adoption of cancer prevention practices such as smoking cessation (Lebovitz et al., 1981). Repetitive notification with appropriate reinforcement may be necessary to confront such psychological barriers to adherence. Education about the benefits of early detection and treatment and postnotification support are necessary components of worker notification strategies (Schulte & Ringen, 1984). Finally, although average levels of psychological distress among exposed workers may not be elevated, a small minority of workers might suffer excessive distress and dysfunction. Physicians should be alert to stress symptoms in these populations, including intrusive thoughts, negative moods, and sleep disruption (Horowitz, 1985). Workers who experience such symptoms might require referrals to special support programs.

FUTURE STUDIES ON THE IMPACT OF CANCER SCREENING

The growing numbers of persons who participate in cancer screening programs underscore the importance of continued research to evaluate the impact of this experience on psychological status and subsequent adherence behavior. One important limitation of the research reviewed here has been the lack of prescreening psychological data. Thus, it is not possible to determine whether persons with positive results or occupational exposures and those in the control groups had equivalent baseline psychological profiles. This is of particular concern because at least one previous study suggests that psychological "responses" observed among women with positive results may be antecedents to screening, rather than the effects of a positive result (Hughes, Royle, Buchanan, & Taylor, 1986). Additionally, differences in subject populations, psychological instruments, and measurement points make it difficult to draw conclusions from this literature. Future studies will be strengthened by utilizing multiple observations, including prior to screening, while anticipating notification, following notification, and during and after diagnostic follow-up. Such studies are essential to identify temporal fluctuations that characterize the coping process and to identify the optimal times for behavioral intervention. In addition, it would be helpful if researchers would use validated scales to permit comparisons of subject populations. It also will be especially important to include adequate numbers of minorities and older adults.

Personality and situational factors that moderate the impact of abnormal findings also should be identified. For example, individual differences in dispositional coping styles have been shown to play an important role in emotional responses and behavior in stressful medical situations (Miller & Mangan, 1983; Lerman, Daly, Masny, Balshem et al., 1994; Scheier, Weintraub, & Carver, 1986). Based on these studies, one would predict that persons with low needs for information or pessimistic coping styles might be more distressed and less likely to adhere to recommended follow-up following notification or screening. The process and content of health communications about positive findings also would be expected to be an important determinant of psychological and behavioral consequences. Previous studies have shown that subtle differences in the framing of risk-related information can have dramatic effects on risk perceptions and health behavior (Wilson, Purdon, & Wallston, 1988; Meyerowitz & Chaiken, 1987). Future studies could examine the possible interacting effects of notification strategies and coping styles on psychological distress and adherence following positive results (Miller & Mangan, 1983). In particular, women who are pessimistic or who have low needs for information may become more anxious when provided with high levels of information about test results and follow-up procedures. Thus, optimal education strategies may be those that tailor the amount and style of information to individual needs.

Helping people who have received abnormal test results to make informed, effective personal decisions also is an important area of study. For example, recent studies have applied techniques from decision analysis to women with early breast cancer (Siminoff & Fetting, 1989; 1991) and to follow-up after an abnormal Pap test (Paskett et al., 1990). Such techniques appear promising. More intervention research is needed to test alternative strategies for informing people about abnormal test results and high-risk status and for encouraging appropriate follow-up (Lerman, Rimer, & Engstrom, 1991).

SUMMARY AND CONCLUSIONS

The studies that have been reviewed here suggest that higher levels of distress may accompany the disclosure of abnormal test results compared with notification of occupational exposures. However, this literature also shows that women with abnormal mammogram results and Pap tests experience only short-term distress. Moreover, the few intervention studies that now have been conducted suggest that simple, potentially cost-effective strategies can be used successfully to reduce distress and improve adherence. The application of these interventions is especially important to assure that those with abnormal results do not drop out of the system for future screening. A note of caution is indicated, however, as some studies suggest that a moderate amount of anxiety may facilitate subsequent screening behavior (Lerman, Trock, Rimer, Boyce, et al., 1991; Kash et al., 1992). Thus, titrating the appropriate dose of anxiety and concern is a challenge. For workers exposed to occupational risks, heightening perceived susceptibility, indeed, may be a requirement for action.

In the next decade, major advances are likely to be made in the technology of cancer screening. This will be coupled with advances in molecular biology and genetic epidemiology that permit finer specification of those who are at risk for cancer. This information may occasionally pose interesting paradoxes. For example, a recent report in the *New England Journal of Medicine* showed that women who carry the gene for ataxia-telangiectasia are especially sensitive to ionizing radiation, despite the fact that they are not affected with the disease. Thus, exposure to diagnostic x-rays probably will increase the risk of breast cancer in these women (Swift, Morrell, Massey, & Chase, 1991). One of the negative sequelae of this report is likely to be increased anxiety about mammography among the vast majority of women who are *not* at risk. Such situations may occur with increasing frequency.

Similarly, advances are being made in the technology of screening for other cancers, such as ovarian cancer and prostate cancer. At this point, little is known about how men and women differ in their reactions to abnormal tests or whether different disease sites generate different concerns. These are questions that should be addressed. Socioeconomic differences also should be considered, not only in terms of response to notification but also in terms of the most appropriate educational programs. Those who embark on cancer screening and risk notification programs should view the communication of abnormal test results as an integral part of the screening process. No screening program should be initiated without a plan that details how the communication of abnormal results and procedures for follow-up will be handled.

Increases in our understanding of the nature of cancer risk and in the utilization of cancer screening pose challenges for those in the psychological sciences. Attention should be paid to characterizing reactions to information about cancer risk and abnormal test results and intervening appropriately with both the screenees and their health providers. The results of these studies also will be applicable to the development of programs for genetic screening for cancer susceptibility (Lerman & Croyle, 1994). Without understanding of and attention to these psychological issues, the potential for cancer screening to reduce morbidity and mortality may go unrealized.

REFERENCES

Alagna, S. W., Morokoff P. J., Bevett J. M., & Reddy, D. M. (1987). Performance of breast self-examination by women at high risk for breast cancer. *Women's Health, 12*(2), 29–46.

Bayer, R. (1986). Notifying workers at risk: The politics of the right-to-know. *American Journal of Public Health, 76,* 1352–1356.

Coon, M., & Polakoff, P. (1982). Legal and ethical dilemmas of worker notification. In J. Lee & W. Rom (Eds.), *Legal and ethical dilemmas in occupational safety and health* (pp. 251–268). Ann Arbor, MI: Ann Arbor Science Publishers.

Dales, L. G., Friedman, G. D., & Collen, M. F. (1979). Evaluating periodic multiphasic health checkups: A controlled trial. *Journal of Chronic Diseases, 32,* 385–404.

Dawson, D. A., & Thompson, G. B. (1990). Breast cancer risk factors and screening: United States, 1987. DHHS Publication (PHS) 90-1500.

Ellman, R., Angeli, N., Christians, A., Moss, S., Chamberlain, J., & Maguire, P. (1989). Psychiatric morbidity associated with screening for breast cancer. *British Journal of Cancer, 60,* 781–784.

Flanders, W. D., & Rothman, K. J. (1982). Occupational risk for laryngeal cancer. *American Journal of Public Health, 72,* 369–372.

Gram, I. T., Lund, E., & Slenker, S. E. (1990). Quality of life following a false positive mammogram. *British Journal of Cancer, 62,* 1018–22.

Greenwald, P., & Sondik, E. (Eds.) (1986). Cancer Control Objectives for the Nation: 1985–2000, Monograph 2, Publication (PHS) 86-2880. Bethesda, MD: National Cancer Institute.

Guzick, D. S. (1978). Efficacy of screening for cervical cancer: A review. *American Journal of Public Health, 68*, 125–134.

Haefner, D. P., Becker, M. H., Janz, N. K., & Rutt, W. M. (1989). Impact of a negative breast biopsy on subsequent breast self-examination practice. *Patient Education and Counseling, 14*, 137–146.

Hoar, S. K., Bang, K. M., Tillett, S., Rodriguez, M., Cantor, K., & Blair, A. (1986). Screening for colorectal cancer and polyps among pattern makers. *Journal of Occupational Medicine, 28*(8), 704–708.

Hornsby, J. L., Sappington, J. T., Mongan, P., Gullen, W., Bono, S., & Altekruse, E. (1985). Risk for bladder cancer: Psychological impact of notification. *Journal of the American Medical Association, 253*(13), 1899–1902.

Horowitz, M. (1985). News of risk as a potential stressor. [Editorial]: *Journal of the American Medical Association, 253*, 1929.

Houts, P. S., & McDougall, V. (1988). Effects of informing workers of their health risks from exposure to toxic materials. *American Journal of Internal Medicine, 13*, 271–279.

Houts, P. S., Wojtkowiak, S. L., Simmonds, M. A., Weinberg, G. B., & Heitjan, D. F. (1991). Using a state cancer registry to increase screening behaviors of sisters and daughters of breast cancer patients. *American Journal of Public Health, 81*(3), 386–388.

Hughes, J. E., Royle, G. T., Buchanan, R., & Taylor, I. (1986). Depression and social stress among patients with benign breast disease. *British Journal of Surgery, 73*, 997–999.

Hutchinson, W. B., Thomas, D. B., Hamlin, W. B., Roth, G. J., Peterson, A. V., & Williams, B. (1980). Risk of breast cancer in women with benign breast disease. *Journal of the National Cancer Institute, 65*(1), 13–20.

Janis, I. L., & Feshbach, S. (1953). Effects of fear-arousing communications. *Journal of Abnormal and Social Psychology, 48*, 78–92.

Kash, K. M., Holland, J. C., Halper, M. S., & Miller, D. G. (1992). Psychological distress and surveillance behaviors of women with a family history of breast cancer. *Journal of the National Cancer Institute, 84*, 24–30.

Kelly, P. T. (1991). *Understanding Breast Cancer Risk.* Philadelphia, PA: Temple University Press.

Lebovitz, A. H., Chahinian, A. P., Gorzynski, J. G., & Holland (1981). Psychological aspects of asbestos-related mesothelioma and knowledge of high risk for cancer. *Cancer Detection and Prevention, 4*, 181–184.

Lerman, C., & Croyle, R. (1994). Psychological issues in genetic testing for breast cancer susceptibility. *Archives of Internal Medicine.* March 28, 154, 609–616.

Lerman, C., Daly, M., Masney, A., & Balshem, A. (1994) Attitudes about genetic testing for breast-ovarian cancer susceptibility. *Journal of Clinical Oncology, 12*(4), 843–850.

Lerman, C., Daly, M., Sands, C., Balshem, A., Lustbader, E., Goldstein, L., James, J., & Engstrom, P. (1993). Mammography adherence and psychological distress among women at risk for breast cancer. *Journal of the National Cancer Institute, 85*(13), 1074–1080.

Lerman, C., Hanjani, P., Caputo, C., Miller, S., Delmoor, E., Nolte, S., & Engstrom, P. (1992). Telephone counseling improves adherence to colposcopy among lower-income minority women. *Journal of Clinical Oncology, 10*(2), 1–4.

Lerman, C., Miller, S., Scarborough, R., Hanjani, P., Nolte, S., & Smith, D. (1991).

Adverse psychologic consequences of positive cytologic cervical screening. *American Journal of Obstetrics and Gynecology, 165,* 658–62.

Lerman, C., Rimer, B., & Engstrom, P. F. (1989). Reducing avoidable cancer mortality through prevention and early detection regimens. *Cancer Research, 49,* 4955–4962.

———. (1991). Cancer risk notification: Psychosocial and ethical implications. *Journal of Clinical Oncology, 9,* 1275–1282.

Lerman, C., Rimer, B., Trock, B., Balshem, A., & Engstrom, P. F. (1990). Factors associated with repeat adherence to breast cancer screening. *Preventive Medicine, 19,* 279–290.

Lerman, C., Ross, E., Boyce, A., McGovern Gorchov, P., McLaughlin, R., Rimer, B., & Engstrom, P. (1992). A randomized trial of psychoeducational materials for women with abnormal mammograms. *American Journal of Public Health, 82,* 729–730.

Lerman, C., Trock, B., Rimer, B., Boyce, A., Jepson, C., & Engstrom, P. (1991). Psychological and behavioral implications of abnormal mammograms. *Annals of Internal Medicine, 114,* 657–661.

Lerman, C., Trock, B., Rimer, B., Jepson, C., Brody, D., & Boyce, A. (1991). Psychological side effects of breast cancer screening. *Health Psychology, 10*(4), 259–267.

Leventhal, H. (1965). Fear communications in the acceptance of preventive health practices. *Bulletin of the New York Academy of Medicine, 41,* 1144–1168.

Mason, T. J., Prorok, P. C., Neeld, W. E., & Vogler, V. (1986). Screening for bladder cancer at the Du Pont Chambers Works: Initial findings. *Journal of Occupational Medicine, 28*(10), 1011–1019.

McDonald, T., Neutens, J., Fischer, L., & Jessee, D. (1989). Impact of cervical intraepithelial neoplasia diagnosis and treatment on self-esteem and body image. *Gynecologic Oncology, 34,* 345–349.

Meyerowitz, B. E., & Chaiken, S. (1987). The effect of message framing on breast self-examination attitudes, intentions, and behavior. *Journal of Personality and Social Psychology, 52*(3), 500–510.

Meyerowitz, B. E., Sullivan, C. D., & Premeau, C. L. (1989). Reactions of asbestos-exposed workers to notification and screening. *American Journal of Internal Medicine, 15,* 463–475.

Miller, S. M., & Mangan, C. E. (1983). Interacting effects of information and coping style in adapting to gynecologic stress: Should the doctor tell all? *Journal of Personal and Social Psychology, 45,* 223–236.

Morris, T., & Greer, S. (1982). Psychological characteristics of women electing to attend a breast screening clinic. *Clinical Oncology, 8,* 113–119.

Nerenz, D., & Leventhal, H. (1983). Self-regulation theory in chronic illness. In T. Burish & L. Bradley (Eds.). *Coping with chronic illness* (pp. 12–37). New York: Academic Press.

Paskett, E. D., White, E., Carter, W. B., & Chu, J. (1990). Improving follow-up after an abnormal pap smear: A randomized controlled trial. *Preventive Medicine, 19,* 630–641.

Reelick, N. F., De Haes, W. F. M., & Schuurman, J. H. (1984). Psychological side-effects of the mass screening on cervical cancer. *Social Science and Medicine, 18*(12), 1089–1093.

Romsaas, E. P., Malec, J. F., Jarenkoski, B. R., Trump, D. L., & Wolberg, W. H.

(1986). Psychological distress among women with breast problems. *Cancer, 57,* 890–895.

Sands, R., Newby, L., & Greenberg, R. (1981). Labeling of health risk in industrial settings. *Journal of Applied Behavioral Science, 17,* 359–374.

Scheier, M. F., Weintraub, J. K., & Carver, C. S. (1986). Coping with stress: Divergent strategies of optimists and pessimists. *Journal of Personality and Social Psychology, 51*(6), 1257–1264.

Schulte, P. A., & Ringen, K. (1984). Notification of workers at high risk: An emerging public health problem. *American Journal of Public Health, 74*(5), 485–491.

Siminoff, L. A., & Fetting, J. H. (1989). Effects of outcome framing on treatment decisions in the real world: Impact of framing on adjuvant breast cancer decisions. *Medical Decision Making, 9,* 135.

————. (1991). Factors affecting decisions for a life-threatening illness: The case of medical treatment of breast cancer. *Social Science and Medicine, 32,* 813–818.

Swift, M., Morrell, D., Massey, R. B., & Chase, C. L. (1991). Incidence of cancer in 161 families affected by ataxia-telangiectasia. *New England Journal of Medicine, 325*(26), 1831–1836.

Tabar, L., & Dean, P. B. (1987). The control of breast cancer through mammography screening: What is the evidence? In E. A. Sickles (Ed.), *The Radiologic Clinics of North America (Breast Imaging)* (pp. 993–1005). Philadelphia: WB Saunders Company.

US Department of Health and Human Services (1989). Fifth annual report on carcinogenesis. Rockville, MD: National Institutes of Health.

Wardle, J., Collins, W., Pernet, A., Whitehead, M., Bourne, H., & Campbell, S. (1993). Psychological impact of screening for familial ovarian cancer. *Journal of the National Cancer Institute, 85,* 653–657.

Weinstein, N. D. (1989). Optimistic biases about personal risk. *Science, 246,* 1232–1233.

Wilkinson, C., Jones, J. M., & McBride, J. (1990). Anxiety caused by abnormal result of cervical smear test: a controlled trial. *British Medical Journal, 300,* 440.

Wilson, D. K., Purdon, S. E., & Wallston, K. A. (1988). Compliance to health recommendations: A theoretical overview of message framing. *Health Education Research, Theory and Practice, 3*(2), 161–171.

Winchester, D. P., Lasky, H. J., Sylvester, J., & Mayer. (1988). A television-promoted mammography screening pilot project in the Chicago metropolitan area. *CA: Cancer Journal for Clinicians, 38*(5), 291–309.

5

Changes in Psychological Distress and HIV Risk-Associated Behavior: Consequences of HIV Antibody Testing?

JOHN B. JEMMOTT, III
CATHERINE A. SANDERSON
SUZANNE M. MILLER

One of the most important advances in efforts to combat the acquired immunodeficiency syndrome (AIDS) has been the development of serological tests for detection of antibodies to human immunodeficiency virus (HIV), which causes the deadly disease. The use of these tests has reduced dramatically the risk of HIV transmission associated with blood transfusions and blood products. In addition to this public health advantage, HIV antibody testing may have significant medical benefits to individuals. Knowledge of seropositivity could lead to further diagnostics, to prophylactic therapies (e.g., zidovudine [AZT]), and to earlier recognition and treatment of AIDS-related illnesses (Coates et al., 1988).

But, as with other risk factor screening regimens (e.g., Croyle & Jemmott, 1991), HIV antibody testing is not simply a technology implemented in a vacuum. HIV antibody testing can have profound social, psychological, and behavioral effects on individuals who are tested. Unfortunately, these effects are currently not well documented. The issue is particularly pressing because of the large numbers of people who are tested. A 1988 National Health Interview Survey indicated

82

that 75% of adults had heard of the HIV antibody test, 17% had been tested (most often as a result of donating blood), and 6% planned to be tested in the upcoming year (Hardy & Dawson, 1990). These figures suggest that approximately 5 million adults may voluntarily seek HIV antibody testing in the next year. Other individuals may undergo mandatory testing, which is required for people seeking to enlist in the military, for immigrants seeking entry into the United States, for federal prisoners, and sometimes for marriage-license and insurance applicants (Kelly & St. Lawrence, 1987).

HIV infection results from exposure to infected blood, semen, or vaginal secretions. Inasmuch as the blood supply in the United States has been screened for HIV antibodies since 1985 (Rugg, MacGowan, Stark, & Swanson, 1991), currently the most common mechanisms of HIV transmission are (a) the sharing of contaminated hypodermic needles and other drug paraphernalia by injection-drug users, (b) the exchange of infected semen, blood, or vaginal secretions during sexual activities, and (c) vertical transmission from infected mothers to their newborns.

HIV antibody testing may ameliorate these remaining mechanisms of transmission. Awareness of HIV-seropositive status might lead individuals to avoid transmitting the virus to others, and awareness of HIV-seronegative status might motivate individuals to make appropriate behavior changes to avoid infection. For instance, the risk of contracting or transmitting HIV might become more salient to individuals as a result of having been tested, and this increased salience might prompt them to adopt behaviors that reduce such risks. On the other hand, there is the possibility that testing may have unintended deleterious consequences. Awareness of HIV-seronegative status might reinforce risky behavior among those who have engaged in such practices by increasing their sense of invulnerability.

It is also important to weigh the emotional impact of awareness of HIV-seropositive status. A positive HIV test result indicates the presence of antibodies to HIV, meaning that the individual has been infected with the virus. A person is HIV seropositive if the results of both repeated enzyme-linked immunoassay (ELISA) tests and a Western blot test are positive. Although individuals who are HIV seropositive may remain asymptomatic for a number of years (Moss et al., 1988), they face the grim prospect of serious illness leading to death. But this is only part of the problem, for AIDS is a stigmatizing condition that many associate with immorality. Consequently, HIV-seropositive individuals may be alienated from friends and family, and they may suffer discrimination in the workplace and from insurance companies and health care personnel (Jemmott, Freleicher, & Jemmott, 1992; Jemmott, Jemmott, & Cruz-Collins, 1992). Indeed, one poll found that 29% of Americans favored a tattoo for anyone testing positive for HIV (Singer, Rogers, & Cocoran, 1987). In this light, it is necessary to consider the possibility that the emotional and psychological devastation associated with knowledge of a positive HIV result may outweigh any potential benefits of testing (Coates et al., 1988), given the fact that a cure is not yet available.

In this chapter, we review critically research related to two main questions that are pertinent to HIV antibody testing. First, what are the emotional consequences of HIV antibody test result? In particular, do positive test results heighten psychological distress? Second, what are the effects of HIV antibody testing on risk-associated behavior? Does notification of a positive test result decrease risk-associated behavior, whereas notification of a negative test result provide a false sense of "immunity" and encourage risky behavior? We used PsychLit and MEDLINE searches to identify relevant articles and also examined references cited in those sources. We excluded studies that examined reactions to HIV antibody test results in patients who were already showing symptoms of AIDS or AIDS-related complex (ARC), case studies, and experimental drug trials on HIV-seropositive individuals.

HIV ANTIBODY TESTING AND PSYCHOLOGICAL DISTRESS

Many people fear being tested for HIV because they expect to feel distress if the results are positive. This expectation has been confirmed by research suggesting negative psychological reactions to such results. Table 5.1 summarizes the studies of the relation of HIV-antibody testing to psychological distress. In one study (Cleary et al., 1988), 29% of the HIV-seropositive blood donors who returned to the New York Blood Center to learn their test results scored at the level for high-risk depression on the Center for Epidemiologic Studies Depression Scale (CES-D), compared with only 13% to 19% of community samples who have scores this high. More than 80% indicated that they were somewhat or very worried or concerned. These results are difficult to interpret, however, because there were no measures of depression prior to testing or depression scores from blood donors who were seronegative. In addition, unlike the majority of subjects in studies of HIV antibody testing, most of these individuals were tested incidentally—donating blood, not being tested for HIV, was their primary goal—and hence presumably they were shocked by their results. The length of time these high level depression scores were sustained is impossible to determine because this study did not include follow-up assessments.

Kaisch and Anton-Culver (1989) also found evidence of psychological distress among HIV-seropositive individuals. In their study, men who were members of homophile organizations in Southern California responded to a mailed survey that included questions about HIV-antibody testing and Institute for Personality and Ability Testing (IPAT) measures of anxiety and depression. The respondents included 30 who said they had received positive results on the HIV antibody test, 55 who said they had received negative results, and 19 who said they did not know their results. Although the study report did not indicate how long the men knew their serostatus, the self-reported HIV-seropositives scored higher on both anxiety and depression than did the self-reported seronegatives. About one third of the seropositive men had clinically elevated levels of anxiety, approximately one half had clinically elevated levels of depression, and about 40% reported thinking about suicide (at some time) after serostatus notification. These results are consistent with the hypothesis that psychological distress follows notification of positive HIV results. The study, however, did not collect any baseline psychological measures prior to antibody testing.

Blaney, Millon, Morgan, Eisdorfer, and Szapocznik (1990) examined psychological distress among 45 healthy HIV-seropositive gay men who had been aware of their serostatus for at least several months and 13 HIV-seronegative gay men who knew their serostatus. The seropositives scored higher than did the seronegatives on the Profile of Mood States (POMS) tension/anxiety, depression, and confusion subscales. However, it should be noted that the seronegatives in the sample were on average below the norms in psychological distress for college students. On average, the HIV-seropositive men scored above college student norms in psychological distress, but below psychiatric outpatient norms.

In their recent report of their study of factors influencing suicide intent in gay and bisexual men, Schneider, Taylor, Hammen, Kemeny, and Dudley (1991) reported data on psychological distress among 778 gay and bisexual men in the Los Angeles site of the Multicenter AIDS Cooperative Study (MACS). Although 27% of the men reported having suicidal ideation in the previous 6 months, there was no difference between the HIV-seropositives and seronegatives. In addition, the two groups did not differ in scores on the Hopelessness scale, POMS total mood disturbance scores, and CES-D depression scores.

Table 5.1. Studies of Psychological Consequences of HIV Antibody Testing

Study	Number	Gender	Race	% Gay/ Bisexual	% IDU	Setting	Design	Major Findings
Antoni, Baggett, et al. (1991)	47	Male	NR	100%	0%	Florida community	Experiment	No serostatus × condition × time interaction on anxiety or depression. Increases in depression were greater among HIV-seropositives in the control condition than among HIV-seropositives in the cognitive-behavioral stress-management condition. Among seronegatives anxiety decreased, whereas among seropositives it increased.
Antoni et al. (1991)	71	Male	71% White 1% Black 14% Hispanic	100%	0%	Florida community	Longitudinal	Seropositives, as compared with seronegatives, scored higher in anxiety and depression at several timepoints but differences were greatest 2 weeks after serostatus notification.
Blaney et al. (1990)	45	Male	64% White 47% Hispanic	100%	NR	Florida cohort study	Cross-sectional	Seropositives scored higher than did seronegatives on the Profile of Mood States (POMS) tension/ anxiety, depression, and confusion subscales

Study	N	Sex	Ethnicity			Setting	Design	Findings
Cleary et al. (1988)	173	78% Male	43% White 32% Black 22% Hispanic	62%	7%	New York City Blood Center	Cross-sectional	29% of HIV-seropositive blood donors scored at the level for high-risk depression on the Center for Epidemiologic Studies Depression Scale (CES-D), compared with only 13% to 19% of community samples who have scores this high.
Doll et al. (1990)	309	Male	93% White 3% Black 3% Hispanic	100%	NR	San Francisco cohort study	Longitudinal	Men who had chosen to learn their HIV serostatus were lower in state anxiety than were those who had chosen not to learn their serosatus. Seropositives were higher in state anxiety than were seronegatives.
Huggins et al. (1991)	56	Male	100% White	100%	NR	Pittsburgh cohort study	Longitudinal	Seropositive, seronegative, and unaware men did not differ in the change in state anxiety and depression from initial assessment to 6 months after notification. However, state anxiety and depression increased in the seropositive group but decreased in the seronegative group from before-notification to 2 weeks after notification. By 6 months after notification, psychological distress returned to baseline in the seropositive group.

(Continued on next page)

Table 5.1. Studies of Psychological Consequences of HIV Antibody Testing (*cont.*)

Study	Number	Gender	Race	% Gay/ Bisexual	% IDU	Setting	Design	Major Findings
Ironson et al. (1991)	36	Male	75% White 3% Black 19% Hispanic	100%	NR	Florida community	Longitudinal	When scores were averaged over all time periods, seropositives were higher in state anxiety than were seronegatives; the difference was greatest at time of serostatus notification.
Kaisch & Anton-Culver (1989)	85	Male	NR	100%	NR	Southern California survey	Longitudinal	Self-reported seropositives scored higher on both anxiety and depression than did self-reported seronegatives. About one third of seropositives had clinical levels of anxiety, about one half had clinical levels of depression, and about 40% had suicidal thoughts (at some time) after serostatus notification.
LaPerriere et al. (1990)	50	Male	74% White 2% Black 20% Hispanic	100%	0%	Florida community	Experiment	Seropositives in the control condition had larger increases in anxiety and depression than did seropositives in the exercise condition and seronegatives in the control and exercise conditions.

| Moulton et al. (1991) | 107 | Male | 97% White | 100% | NR | San Francisco General Hospital cohort study | Longitudinal | 12 months after serostatus notification (but not 2 weeks, 3 months, or 6 months after notification), notified seropositives reported greater increases in total distress than did unnotified seropositives. However, the notified seropositives had a *smaller* increase in hopelessness 2 weeks after notification than did the not-notified seropositives. Seronegatives who chose to learn their serostatus had significantly greater decreases in hopelessness at 2 weeks, 3 months, and 12 months after notification and marginally significantly greater decreases 6 months after notification. However, differences between notified and not-notified seronegatives on anxiety and total distress were not significant at any timepoint. |

(Continued on next page)

Table 5.1. Studies of Psychological Consequences of HIV Antibody Testing (*cont.*)

Study	Number	Gender	Race	% Gay/ Bisexual	% IDU	Setting	Design	Major Findings
Ostrow et al. (1989)	474	Male	93% White	100%	NR	Chicago cohort study	Longitudinal	Seropositives who chose to learn their test results showed significantly greater increases in obsessive-compulsive and depression symptom scores from before notification to 1 year after notification than did seropositive men who chose not to learn their test results; among seronegatives, in contrast, there were no significant differences in changes in psychological distress between those who chose to learn and those who chose not to learn their test results.
Perry et al. (1993)	328	86% Male	79% White	72%	10%	New York City clinic	Longitudinal	The seropositives and the seronegatives did not differ in state anxiety, depression, or clinical ratings of depression one year after notification. Both serostatus groups had lower scores on these measures one year after notification as compared with initial values (prior to testing).

| Perry et al. (1991) | 307 | 87% Male | 76% White | 65% | 15% | New York City clinic | Longitudinal | Among the seropositives, mean distress measures decreased significantly at the 3-month follow-up after stress prevention training and did not change after the other two interventions. Among the seronegatives, mean distress measures decreased significantly after all three interventions. |
| Perry, Jacobsberg, & Fishman (1990) | 301 | 81% Male | 73% White 13% Black 10% Hispanic | 66% | 12% | New York City clinic | Longitudinal | In the sample as a whole, the percentage of subjects who reported having suicidal ideation in the previous week declined from 2 weeks before serostatus notification to 1 week and 2 months after notification. A serostatus × time interaction indicated that the rate of decline was faster among seronegatives as compared with seropositives. |

(Continued on next page)

Table 5.1. Studies of Psychological Consequences of HIV Antibody Testing (*cont.*)

Study	Number	Gender	Race	% Gay/Bisexual	% IDU	Setting	Design	Major Findings
Perry, Jacobsberg, Weiler et al. (1990)	218	80% Male	73% White 12% Black 11% Hispanic	67%	12%	New York City clinic	Longitudinal	The seronegatives and the seropositives did not differ in state anxiety, depression, global distress, or clinical ratings of depression 2 weeks before notification or 10 weeks after notification. Both serostatus groups had significant reductions in state anxiety, depression, and global distress 10 weeks after notification as compared with initial values.
Schneider et al. (1991)	778	Male	91% White	100%		Los Angeles cohort study	Cross-sectional	Seropositives and seronegatives did not differ in suicidal ideation in the past 6 months, CES-D depression, POMS total mood disturbance, or hopelessness.

Note: IDU = injection-drug user; NR = not reported.

None of these studies examined data on psychological distress measured prior to notification of HIV serostatus. Hence, it is equally plausible that knowledge of HIV seropositivity was associated with an increase in psychological distress and that HIV-seropositive individuals, irrespective of knowledge of serostatus, are higher in psychological distress. Prospective studies allow us to examine this issue more precisely. One study was conducted using a heterogeneous sample (gay/bisexual men, intravenous [IV] drug users, heterosexuals with partners at risk) of physically asymptomatic adults. The subjects received before and after HIV antibody test counseling and were evaluated 2 weeks before HIV serostatus notification and 2 and 10 weeks after notification. In one report (Perry, Jacobsberg, Fishman, Weiler, et al., 1990), data from 218 subjects indicated that seronegatives (n = 179) and seropositives (n = 39) did not differ in state anxiety (Spielberger State Anxiety Inventory, SAI), depression (Beck Depression Inventory), global distress (Brief Symptom Inventory, BSI) or clinical ratings of depression (Hamilton Depression Rating Scale, HDRS) 2 weeks before notification or 10 weeks after notification. Both serostatus groups had significant reductions in state anxiety, depression, and global distress at 10 weeks after notification as compared with initial values. The seronegatives also declined in clinical ratings of depression 10 weeks after notification, whereas the seropositives' scores did not change significantly. Similarly, in another study using the same measures and type of sample, Perry et al. (1993) found that knowledge of serostatus did not increase psychiatric morbidity at a one-year follow-up.

In a third report, Perry, Jacobsberg, and Fishman (1990) focused on the issue of suicidal ideation, presenting data from 301 subjects. Seropositives and seronegatives did not differ significantly in rates of suicidal thoughts 2 weeks before serostatus notification. However, the percentage of subjects who reported having suicidal ideation in the previous week declined significantly over time, and the pattern of decline was significantly different for seronegatives and seropositives. Among the 252 seronegatives, reports of suicidal ideation in the past week decreased from 30.6% prior to notification to 17.1% at 1 week and 15.9% at 2 months after notification. In contrast, among the 49 seropositives, suicidal ideation did not change from before notification (when 28.6% reported such ideation) to 1 week after notification (when 27.1% gave such responses). However, suicidal ideation was significantly reduced at the 2-month follow-up, when 16.3% reported such thoughts.

.Other research has found few long-lived psychological effects of HIV testing as well. Seropositives sometimes manifest an increase in anxiety at notification, but their scores return to baseline as little as 3 weeks later. For example, Ironson et al. (1990) measured psychological distress in the 5-week periods preceding and following notification of serostatus among 46 gay men. When scores were averaged across all time periods, the seropositive men scored significantly higher on the state version of the State-Trait Anxiety Inventory than did the seronegative men. However, this difference was greatest at time of notification of serostatus. Immediately after notification of serostatus, mean state anxiety of the seropositives was near values listed for neuropsychiatric patients with depressive reaction, but it returned to baseline values by 3 weeks after notification, values that were comparable to the norms for college men.

Using a similar design, Antoni et al. (1991) measured psychological distress in the 5-week periods preceding and following serostatus notification among 71 gay men. Although the investigators did not indicate whether there was an interaction between serostatus and time, they reported that seropositives, as compared with seronegatives, had higher POMS anxiety scores at 72 hours before notification and 2 weeks, 3 weeks, and 5 weeks after notification. The greatest difference was at the 2 weeks' post-notification assessment. Seropositives also scored higher in POMS depression than did seronegatives at every timepoint, with the largest disparity at the 2 weeks' post-notification timepoint. The state version of the State-Trait Anxiety Inventory (STAI) was administered immediately after notification, as well as at the other timepoints. As compared with seronegatives, seropositives were more anxious at 72 hours before notification, immediately after notification, and 2 weeks after notification. This discrepancy was largest at the time of serostatus notification. By 5 weeks after notification, scores on all three measures had returned to baseline levels in both groups.

Huggins, Elmon, Baker, Forrester, and Lyter (1991) studying gay men found significant serostatus × time interactions that were consistent with the pattern of findings obtained by Ironson et al. (1990) and Antoni et al. (1991). State anxiety and depression rose among the 22 seropositive men but decreased among the 22 seronegative men from before notification to 2 weeks after notification. At a 6 months' post-notification assessment, anxiety and depression remained decreased in the seronegative group and returned to baseline in the seropositive group.

Receipt versus Nonreceipt of HIV Antibody Test Results

Taken together, the results of these studies suggest that although anxiety increases in seropositives as compared with seronegatives, the increase is relatively short lived. In the research reviewed thus far, the subjects knew their serostatus and the contrast was between the reactions of seropositives and those of seronegatives. However, another way to examine the effects of serostatus is to examine (a) whether distress differs significantly among seropositives who are notified of their serostatus as compared with seropositives who are not notified of their status and (b) whether distress differs significantly among seronegatives who are notified of their serostatus as compared with seronegatives who are not notified of their serostatus. Four studies have considered the effects of serostatus by contrasting notified and not-notified individuals.

The results of a study by Ostrow et al. (1989) on 585 gay men who had been tested for HIV antibodies as part of a cohort study suggested significant effects of serostatus notification among seropositives but not among seronegatives. All of the subjects completed the Hopkins Symptom Checklist administered prior to disclosure of serostatus and about 1 year later, after disclosure. Although Ostrow et al. (1989) did not indicate whether the serostatus × notification interaction was significant, they did report that seropositive men who chose to learn their test results showed significantly greater increases in obsessive-compulsive and depression symptoms than did seropositive men who chose not to learn their test results. In contrast, seronegatives who did or did not choose to learn their test results did not differ significantly in changes over time in psychological distress.

Doll et al. (1990) studied 181 homosexual and bisexual men in the San Francisco city clinic cohort. The subjects completed the Zung Depression Scale and the state version of the Spielberger State-Trait Anxiety Inventory an average of 17 months (range, 4 to 28 months) after they chose to learn or not to learn their HIV serostatus. Because state anxiety and depression scores were available only after the men had learned of their antibody test results, only cross-sectional analyses could be performed. No effects emerged on depression scores. However, seropositives were significantly higher in state anxiety than were seronegatives. In addition, the men who had chosen to learn their HIV serostatus were significantly lower in state anxiety than were those who had chosen not to learn their serostatus. These results suggest that not knowing one's serostatus may be more anxiety provoking than knowing it. Unfortunately, Doll et al. did not indicate whether the effects of notification were different among seronegatives and seropositives. Unclear, for instance, is whether reduced distress among seronegatives who learned they were uninfected accounts for the lower distress among those notified of serostatus.

The previously mentioned study of Huggins et al. (1991) also compared notified and not-notified gay and bisexual men. The results revealed that changes over time on the state version of the State-Trait Anxiety Scale and the Beck Depression Inventory from before notification to 6 months after notification were not significantly different among seronegatives, seropositives, and not-notified men. Unfortunately, like Doll et al. (1990), Huggins et al. (1991) did not separate the unaware group into unaware seropositives and unaware seronegatives.

A study by Moulton, Stempel, Bacchetti, Temoshok, and Moss (1991) examined 107 homosexual men in San Francisco. The subjects completed the Profile of Mood States (POMS), the abbreviated Taylor Manifest Anxiety Scale, and the Beck Hopelessness Scale about 2 weeks prior to serostatus notification and 2 weeks, 3 months, 6 months, and 12 months after notification. Analyses revealed that 12 months after serostatus notification (but not earlier) notified seropositives reported significantly greater increases in POMS total distress than did the seropositives who were not notified. However, there were no significant differences between notified and not-notified seropositives in changes in anxiety at any of the follow-ups. Surprisingly, the notified seropositives had a *smaller* increase in hopelessness 2 weeks after notification than did the not-notified seropositives. No other differences between notified and not-notified seropositives were significant. Among seronegatives, there was some evidence of relief. Those who chose to learn their serostatus had significantly greater decreases in hopelessness at 2 weeks, 3 months, and 12 months after notification and marginally significantly greater decreases at 6 months after notification. However, differences between notified and not-notified seronegatives on anxiety and total distress were not significant at any timepoint. Because Moulton et al. (1991) did not indicate whether the serostatus × notification interaction was significant, it is unclear whether serostatus notification had a significantly less distressful effect on seronegatives as compared with seropositives.

Although these four studies collected data bearing on the effects of notification of HIV serostatus, they do not provide a clear-cut resolution of the issue. The results were inconsistent. One study suggested that notified seropositives were higher in distress than were not-notified seropositives but that there were no differences between notified and not-notified seronegatives. Another study found only weak evidence of this higher distress in notified seropositives but reported some evidence of reduced distress among notified seronegatives compared with not-notified seronegatives. To untangle these effects, future studies should distinguish between aware seropositives and aware seronegatives, examine interactions between serostatus and knowledge of serostatus, and employ prospective designs. As in other medical contexts, effects of notification may be moderated by individual difference variables such as information-seeking style (Miller, Combs, & Stoddard, 1989).

Interventions to Reduce Distress Associated with Serostatus Notification

A final issue that has been explored with respect to the psychological distress associated with HIV antibody testing is the effectiveness of interventions designed to improve emotional adjustment in individuals who have a positive antibody test result. Two well-controlled studies have provided data on this issue. One focused on reducing distress after serostatus notification by augmenting the standard posttest counseling. A second focused on short-circuiting distress by intervening prior to serostatus notification.

Perry, Jacobsberg, Fishman, et al. (1990) tested the effects of stress-prevention interventions of self-reported anxiety, depression, fear of getting AIDS, and fear of having infected others among 218 adults. After posttest counseling, the subjects were randomly assigned to one of three conditions: (a) standard practice, which involved only before and after HIV antibody test counseling; (b) six weekly sessions of cognitive-behavioral stress-prevention training, which began the week after notification and included methods of relaxation and reframing dysfunctional thoughts; or (c) three weekly psychoeducational sessions that were imparted by interactive video. Multivariate analyses revealed no significant differences among the intervention conditions in changes in psychological distress from 2 weeks prior to notification to 1 week and 2 months after notification, nor was there a significant interaction between intervention condition and serostatus on such changes. However, in another study on the effects of interventions on emotional distress, these authors (Perry et al., 1991) found that mean distress measures were significantly lower at the three-month follow-up among the 204 HIV seronegatives after all three interventions, and among the 103 HIV seropositives following the stress prevention training. Distress did not change following the standard counseling or the interactive video sessions among those who were seropositive.

In a separate article, Perry, Jacobsberg, & Fishman (1990) reported additional data from this ongoing study. This report centered on the effects of stress-prevention interventions on suicidal ideation among 301 adults who had undergone HIV antibody testing. Consistent with the initial report, analyses revealed no significant effects of the intervention nor any interactions between type of intervention and serosta-tus or time. As Perry, Jacobsberg, and Fishman (1990) have suggested, the fact that the interventions were aimed at chronic distress rather than acute distress may explain, at least in part, the statistically nonsig-nificant effect of the interventions in 2 studies. In addition, because participants were not selected on the basis of heightened posttesting distress, it is possible that negative results reflect a floor effect.

LaPerriere et al. (1990) and Antoni, Baggett et al. (1991) recently tested the effects of interventions to short-circuit the acute emotional distress associated with notification of positive HIV serostatus. Prior to being tested for HIV antibodies, asymptomatic gay men were as-signed randomly to an aerobic exercise training program, a cognitive-behavioral stress-management program, or an assessment-only control condition. The men in the aerobic exercise training condition partici-pated in 5 weeks of three weekly 45-minute exercise sessions on a bicycle ergometer. Those in the cognitive-behavioral stress-manage-ment condition met twice weekly for 10 weeks in groups of four to six men led by two pre-doctoral students in clinical psychology. LaPerriere et al. (1990) presented data on emotional distress experi-enced 72 hours before serostatus notification and 1 week after notifica-tion among 50 men in the exercise and control conditions. Significant group × time interactions indicated that the HIV seropositives in the control condition had significantly larger increases in anxiety and depression (as measured by the POMS) than did the seropositives in the exercise condition, the seronegatives in the control condition, and the seronegatives in the exercise condition.

Antoni, Baggett et al. (1991) presented data comparing emotional distress among 47 men in the cognitive-behavioral stress-management and control conditions. The interaction of serostatus, condition, and time was not significant on POMS anxiety or depression scores, which indicates that the cognitive-behavioral stress-management interven-tion did not cause a significantly greater reduction in distress among seropositives than among seronegatives. There was an interaction be-tween condition and time on depression (but not anxiety) considering the HIV-seropositive men only. Increases in depression were greater for the HIV-seropositive men in the control condition than for the HIV-seropositive men in the cognitive-behavioral stress-management condition. As in other studies (Antoni et al., 1991; Huggins et al., 1991; Ironson et al., 1990), results showed that anxiety decreased among seronegatives, but increased among seropositives.

Although the results of this study are suggestive, it is not possible to judge whether the exercise and the cognitive behavioral interventions were differentially effective. Moreover, the division of the sample would also seem to have reduced the statistical power of tests of intervention effects, which is particularly problematic given the relatively small sample sizes. In addition, intervention effects might have been stronger had individuals with vulnerable profiles been targeted. Nevertheless, the use of an experimental design with random assignment to conditions is an important strength of this study as well as the Perry and associates' study.

HIV ANTIBODY TESTING AND RISK-ASSOCIATED BEHAVIOR

Table 5.2 summarizes the results of studies on the relation of HIV antibody testing to HIV risk–associated behavior. Studies of the behavioral consequences of HIV antibody testing can be divided into three types: (a) studies comparing individuals whose test result was positive with those whose test result was negative; (b) studies comparing tested individuals with individuals who were not tested; and (c) studies of tested individuals comparing those who received their test results with those who did not receive their test results. We will review each of these, in turn.

Seropositives versus Seronegatives

Individuals who learn they are HIV seropositive may well decrease their risk behavior compared with those who learn they are HIV seronegative. Five studies explored this issue. Schechter et al. (1988) collected data on 361 gay and bisexual men, of whom 130 were seropositive, before disclosure of HIV test results and at a follow-up about 28 months after disclosure. Considering the sample as a whole, there were substantial declines in the self-reported number of annual sexual partners from before disclosure to after disclosure. This decline was not significantly different among the men who learned they were HIV seropositive as compared with those who learned they were HIV seronegative. A more fine-grained analysis performed at the follow-up revealed the HIV-seronegative individuals were less likely to practice receptive anal sex with casual partners than with regular partners; for the HIV-seropositive individuals, type of partner did not matter. One interpretation of these results is that subsequent to testing, the HIV-seronegative individuals became more selective about the partners with whom they engaged in receptive anal intercourse. However, because no distinction was drawn between casual and regular partners in the baseline assessments, it is possible that the HIV-seronegatives

Table 5.2. Studies of Behavioral Consequences of HIV Antibody Testing

Study	Number	Gender	Race	% Gay Men	% IDU	Setting	Design	Major Findings
Coates et al. (1987)	502	Male	91% White	100%	NR	San Francisco cohort study	Longitudinal	A greater percentage of untested as compared with seropositive and seronegative men reported engaging in unprotected insertive anal intercourse after notification; before notification, the groups had reported significantly higher rates of unprotected insertive anal intercourse and had not differed in the rate of unprotected insertive anal intercourse.
Dawson et al. (1991)	502	Male	NR	100%	NR	England survey	Cross-sectional	The men who reported they had been tested engaged in more anal intercourse in previous month than did those who reported they had not been tested. Among the men who reported being tested, there were no significant differences between seropositives and seronegatives in self-reported anal intercourse or condom use in the previous month.

| Doll et al. (1990) | 309 | Male | 93% White 3% Black 3% Hispanic | 100% | NR | San Francisco cohort study | Longitudinal | There were significant declines in receptive and insertive anal intercourse and anal intercourse with both steady and nonsteady partners. However, these declines were independent of HIV serostatus, awareness of serostatus, and the interaction of serostatus and awareness of serostatus. Seropositives had a higher risk index for insertive anal intercourse with casual partners. There was no relationship between length of time since learning of HIV serostatus and persistence of high-risk behavior. |

(Continued on next page)

Table 5.2. Studies of Behavioral Consequences of HIV Antibody Testing (*cont.*)

Study	Number	Gender	Race	% Gay Men	% IDU	Setting	Design	Major Findings
Fox et al. (1987)	1,001	Male	95% White	100%	NR	Baltimore-Washington cohort study	Longitudinal	The aware HIV-seropositive men showed a greater decrease in number of sexual partners with whom they had receptive anal intercourse and the number of sexual partners with whom they had insertive anal intercourse than did the men who were unaware of whether they were seronegative or seropositive. In addition, compared with unaware men, the aware HIV-seronegative men showed a smaller decrease in total number of sexual partners, number of sexual partners with whom they had receptive anal intercourse, and the number of sexual partners with whom they had insertive anal intercourse.

| Frazer et al. (1988) | 318 | Male | NR | 100% | NR | Brisbane, Australia, sample | Cross-sectional | Insertive anal intercourse in the previous 6 months was significantly less common among the aware seropositives than among the unaware seropositives. For seronegatives, however, awareness of HIV serostatus was unrelated to frequency of anal intercourse. A separate analysis was done on the 208 subjects who reported anal intercourse at least once within the previous 3 months. The men who had been tested previously were marginally ($p=.06$) more likely to have used a condom during anal intercourse in the previous 3 months than were those who had not been tested. Those who had been tested and were seropositive were significantly more likely to use a condom always when having anal intercourse than were those who previously had been shown to be negative. Condom use did not differ between those who had previously received negative HIV test results and those who had not been tested. |

(Continued on next page)

Table 5.2. Studies of Behavioral Consequences of HIV Antibody Testing (*cont.*)

Study	Number	Gender	Race	% Gay Men	% IDU	Setting	Design	Major Findings
Huggins et al. (1991)	56	Male	100% White	100%	NR	Pittsburgh cohort study	Longitudinal	Although the sample as a whole showed a significant decrease in anal intercourse as a passive partner over 6 months, the amount of decrease was not significantly different among the seropositives, seronegatives, and men who did not learn their serostatus.
Landis et al. (1992)	235	67% Male	44% Black	17%	12%	North Carolina health department	Longitudinal	No significant net change in high-risk behavior among the 24% who completed the one-year follow-up.
McCusker et al. (1988)	257	Male	97% White	100%	NR	Boston cohort study	Longitudinal	There were substantial declines in the number of casual homosexual partners and the number of anogenital partners (insertive and receptive) over the time period, but no effects of serostatus or knowledge of serostatus. A multiple regression analysis on insertive anogenital contact at the 1-year follow-up revealed that

| Ostrow et al. (1989) | 474 | Male | 93% White | 100% | Chicago cohort study | NR | Longitudinal | seropositives who knew their serostatus declined more and seropositives who did not know declined less than did others. Among men who reported some unprotected anogenital contact at the initial visit, men who became aware of a positive result were less likely to continue insertive contact without a condom than were seropositive men unaware of their result. Among seronegative men, in contrast, those aware of their result were somewhat *more* likely to continue this practice.

Although there was an overall decrease in sexual behavior, HIV antibody test disclosure—whether of a positive or negative test result—did not influence sexual behavior change over the 1-year time period. |

(*Continued on next page*)

105

Table 5.2. Studies of Behavioral Consequences of HIV Antibody Testing (*cont.*)

Study	Number	Gender	Race	% Gay Men	% IDU	Setting	Design	Major Findings
Schechter et al. (1988)	361	Male	NR	100%	NR	Vancouver cohort study	Longitudinal	Substantial declines in the self-reported number of annual sexual partners from before to after disclosure. However, this decline was not significantly different among the men who learned they were HIV seropositive as compared with those who learned they were HIV seronegative. HIV-seronegative individuals were less likely to practice receptive anal sex with casual partners than with regular partners, whereas for the HIV-seropositive individuals, type of partner did not matter. Frequency of condom use with regular partners and with casual partners was markedly higher at follow-up than was the frequency of condom use, ignoring type of partner at baseline. However, the HIV-seronegative men, as compared with HIV-seropositive men, were more likely to report never using condoms during anal intercourse with casual partners.

Source	N	Gender	Ethnicity			Sample	Design	Findings
Van Griensven et al. (1988)	746	Male	NR	100%	NR	Amsterdam cohort study	Longitudinal	Although significance levels were not provided, in the sample as a whole there was a decline in number of sexual partners. The decline among the seropositives was greater than that among the seronegatives.
Van Griensven et al. (1989)	307	Male	NR	100%	NR	Amsterdam cohort study	Longitudinal	Among seropositives, the percent who engaged in insertive anal intercourse with nonsteady partners remained constant, while among seronegatives and untested, the percent who engaged in receptive anal intercourse decreased. Seropositives were more likely to use condoms during insertive anal intercourse with their nonsteady and steady partners than those who are seronegative or untested.
Vanichseni et al. (1992)	601	95% Male	99% Thai	NR	100%	Thailand clinic sample	Cross-sectional	HIV seropositives reported higher levels of safer sex and condom use with primary partners compared to seronegatives and untested. A greater percentage of seropositives with regular partners reported using condoms at least some of the time with that partner in the previous six months.

(Continued on next page)

Table 5.2. Studies of Behavioral Consequences of HIV Antibody Testing (*cont.*).

Study	Number	Gender	Race	% Gay Men	% IDU	Setting	Design	Major Findings
Watkins et al. (1993)	158	77% Male	63% Black	0	100%	Philadelphia methadone clinic	Cross-sectional	Being HIV seropositive was associated with an increased probability of using a condom.
Wenger et al. (1991)	186	67% Male	88% Black	0%		Los Angeles STD clinic sample	Experiment	Although both intervention and control conditions showed a decrease in reported number of sexual partners, the degree of decrease was not significantly different between conditions. In the intervention condition, as compared with the control condition, there was a greater increase in the percentage of subjects who had avoided vaginal or anal intercourse without a condom with their most recent sexual partner and a significantly greater increase in the percentage of subjects who had asked their sexual partners about the partner's HIV serostatus.

Study	N	Gender	Race			Setting	Design	Findings
Wenger et al. (1992)	435	72% Female	61% White	0	NR	University student health center sample	Experiment	Subjects in the education plus testing group questioned their sexual partners about their HIV serostatus more. No consistent differences among the three groups in number of sexual partners or use of condoms were found at the six-month follow-up.
Wiktor et al. (1990)	146	Male	98% White	100%	NR	New York/ Washington, DC, and Copenhagen/ Aarhus cohort studies	Longitudinal	Among HIV seropositives, HIV seronegatives, and those who did not know their serostatus, there were no significant differences in self-reported anal intercourse, number of sexual partners, or condom use.
Zenilman et al. (1992)	1972	78% Male	98% Black	12	25	Baltimore STD clinic	Longitudinal	A greater percentage of HIV seronegatives showed evidence of a STD after testing and counseling in the follow-up period.

Note: IDU = injection-drug user; NR = not reported; STD = sexually transmitted disease.

were less likely to practice receptive anal sex with casual partners prior to as well as following testing.

Schechter et al. also examined condom use. Overall, frequency of condom use with regular partners and with casual partners was markedly higher following serostatus notification than was the frequency of condom use, ignoring type of partner at baseline. As compared with their HIV-seropositive counterparts at follow-up, HIV-seronegative men were more likely to report never using condoms during receptive anal intercourse with casual partners. It is possible that a subset of seronegatives inferred that they were protected from being infected and that this served as a disincentive to behavior change. On the other hand, frequency of condom use during receptive anal intercourse with casual partners was not assessed at the initial assessment. Hence, it is unclear whether seronegatives failed to increase their condom use with such partners specifically and whether the degree of change differed significantly from that among seropositives.

Van Griensven et al. (1988) also examined the sexual behavior of gay men who were notified of their HIV serostatus. The subjects, 746 gay men living in and around Amsterdam, the Netherlands, were tested for HIV (31% were positive) and surveyed at three consecutive 6-month intervals. They were informed of their HIV serostatus after they completed the baseline questionnaire. Although significance levels were not provided, consistent with the findings of Schechter et al. (1988), Van Griensven et al. (1988) reported that in the sample as a whole there was a decline in number of sexual partners. In contrast to Schechter et al., however, Van Griensven et al. also reported that the decline among the seropositives was greater than that among the seronegatives.

A study of intravenous drug users (Watkins et al., 1993) also suggested that seropositive individuals engaged in less risky sexual behavior as compared to those who were seronegative. Seventy-eight percent of HIV seropositives reported using condoms the last time they engaged in intercourse while only 26% of those who were HIV negative reported using condoms. A logistic regression analysis also found that HIV seropositive subjects were 10.6 times more likely to use a condom than those who were HIV seronegative, controlling for age, race, and gender.

Similarly, Zenilman et al. (1992) matched 868 HIV seropositive STD clinic patients with 1104 HIV seronegatives to examine the effect of HIV testing on STD infection. Although the results of this study are somewhat difficult to interpret (due to the smaller percentage of seronegatives who returned to the clinic and whose records were available), the findings indicate that a greater percentage of those who were HIV seronegative showed evidence of infection with an STD during the follow-up period (ranging from 6 months to 23 months). These studies (Van Griensven et al., 1988; Watkins et al., 1993; Zenilman et al., 1992) provide some evidence that individuals who learn they are HIV seropositive may decrease their risk behavior compared to those who learn they are HIV seronegative.

One study, however, found no changes in high-risk sexual behavior as a result of HIV testing (Landis et al., 1992). Landis and colleagues (1992) interviewed 235 people at 2 anonymous HIV testing sites in North Carolina, and asked them to return for a follow-up interview one-year later. Of the 24% who did complete a follow-up interview, there were no significant changes in high-risk sexual behavior as a function of HIV serostatus. It is difficult to draw conclusions from this study, however, given the low return rate and potential selection bias in who returns for the follow-up.

Tested versus Untested Individuals

Six studies have investigated behavioral reactions to HIV antibody testing by comparing tested individuals with individuals who were not tested. Coates, Morin, and McKusick (1987) reported data on 502 gay and bisexual men who were surveyed each November from 1984 (before testing was available) until 1986 (after testing was available) regarding their sexual behavior in the past month. As of November 1986, 41% of the men had been tested for HIV antibodies. Of these, 99 were HIV seropositive, 77 were HIV seronegative, and 8 declined to reveal their serostatus. In the sample as a whole, the posttesting rates of unprotected insertive anal intercourse were generally lower than were the rates prior to testing. The percentage reporting unprotected insertive anal intercourse in the preceding months did not significantly differ among seropositives (48%), seronegatives (41%), and untested individuals (49%) prior to testing. After testing, however, the groups did differ significantly in unprotected insertive anal intercourse in the previous month. About 12% of seropositives, 18% of seronegatives, and 27% of untested individuals reported this behavior. This suggests that antibody testing, regardless of the outcome, may be associated with a reduction in risk-associated sexual behavior.

Unfortunately, the investigators did not report whether the degree of decrease in unprotected insertive anal intercourse was significantly different among the groups. The fact that groups differ at one point in time but not at another does not establish that the groups differ significantly in degree of change. Of particular interest are comparisons between tested and not-tested individuals and between HIV-seropositives and HIV-seronegatives. Inspection of the data suggests that it was the seropositives specifically, rather than tested individuals per se, who changed the most. The reduction in the percentage who engaged in unprotected insertive anal intercourse was greater among seropositives (-36%) than among the seronegatives (-23%) and untested individuals (-22%), who did not differ. However, it is unclear whether these numerical differences are statistically significant.

Van Griensven and colleagues (Van Griensven et al., 1989), however, do provide some evidence that seropositives are more likely to report a decrease in risky sexual behavior. The subjects in this study (some of whom are also included in the study by Van Griensven et al., 1988) include 118 seronegatives, 75 seropositives, and 114 untested gay men in The Netherlands. Among seropositives, the percentage who engaged in active anal intercourse with nonsteady partners remained constant, while among seronegatives and untested individuals, the percentage who engaged in passive anal intercourse with casual partners decreased significantly. Seropositives were, however, significantly more likely to use condoms during insertive intercourse with their nonsteady and steady sexual partners than were seronegatives and untested individuals during receptive anal intercourse with these partners. This study suggests that seropositives are attempting to engage in safer sexual behavior, by using condoms during insertive intercourse, although they are not decreasing their frequency of this behavior.

Similarly, in a study of 601 intravenous drug users in Thailand, Vanichseni et al. (1992) found that HIV testing was associated with higher levels of safer sex and contraceptive use with regular partners. In this study, 56% of the 73 self-reported seropositives used condoms at least some of the time with their regular partners, as compared to only 28% of the seronegatives (N = 148) and 20% of those not tested (N = 336). Furthermore, 89% of the seropositives reported using some type of contraceptive with regular partners while only 72% of the seronegatives and 59% of the untested individuals reported the use of contraceptives.

In contrast, one study has revealed scant evidence that testing is associated with decreased risky sexual activity (Dawson, Fitzpatrick, McLean, Hart, and Boulton, 1991). The subjects, 502 men who reported having sex with another man in the previous 5 years, were recruited from four areas of England. About one half of the men reported they had been tested for HIV antibodies. Of the tested men, 12% indicated they were seropositive, 83% indicated they were seronegative, and 5% indicated they had not yet received their test results. When queried about their sexual behavior in the previous month, the men who reported they had been tested were *more* likely to have had receptive anal intercourse with a casual partner, receptive anal sex without a condom, and insertive anal sex with a regular partner than were those who reported they had not been tested. There were no significant differences between seropositives and seronegatives in self-reported anal intercourse or condom use in the previous month. These results suggest the disturbing conclusion that testing does not reduce risky sexual behavior. However, the study did not assess sexual behavior prior to HIV antibody testing. Accordingly, it is impossible to determine whether the degree of change in sexual behavior varied between those who were and were not tested, or between HIV-seropositive and HIV-seronegative individuals.

One threat to the internal validity of studies that compared tested and not-tested individuals is that differences that emerge may be behavioral correlates of the decision to undergo testing rather than effects of testing. For example, the individuals who decided to be tested might have been committed to changing their behavior before they were tested. For them, testing may have been part of a more general safer behavior agenda. A recent experiment by Wenger, Linn, Epstein, and Shapiro (1991) ruled out this alternative explanation by randomly assigning subjects to be tested or not tested. The 186 subjects were predominantly low-income, black, and heterosexual, and had been recruited at a sexually transmitted disease (STD) clinic. They were given information and counseling about HIV/AIDS, including information about safe and unsafe sexual practices. The participants were then assigned randomly to the intervention condition, which received HIV antibody testing, or the control condition, which received a list of free HIV testing sites. All participants completed a pretest measure prior to antibody testing in the intervention group; those in the intervention group received antibody test results 2 weeks later; and all subjects completed the posttest measure 6 weeks later. All of the tested subjects were found to be seronegative.

The subjects in the two conditions showed a comparable decrease in reported number of sexual partners. However, there was a greater increase in the percentage of subjects in the intervention condition who had avoided vaginal or anal intercourse without a condom with their most recent sexual partner. In addition, there was a significantly greater increase in the percentage of subjects who had asked their sexual partners about the partner's HIV serostatus in the intervention condition than in the control condition. These changes are particularly impressive given that all of the intervention subjects received negative results. Testing for HIV, coupled with counseling, may lead to a reduction in risky behavior, even if the results are negative, compared with counseling alone, at least for individuals attending a STD clinic.

In a replication of this study with 435 heterosexual college students, however, Wenger et al. (1992) found no consistent differences at the 6-month follow-up in the number of sexual partners or in the use of condoms. Students who received HIV testing coupled with education reported questioning their sexual partners about their HIV serostatus more than those who received education alone or those in the control group, but this difference was not found in patterns of risky behavior.

Receipt versus Nonreceipt of HIV Antibody Results

Seven studies have compared tested individuals who chose to receive their test results with those who chose not to receive their test results. For example, Wiktor et al. (1990) administered questionnaires regarding HIV serostatus and sexual practices to 134 homosexual men from a prospective cohort study of AIDS risk in New York City and Washington, DC, and 130 homosexual men from a similar cohort in Copenhagen and Aarhus, Denmark. The participants, all of whom had been tested for HIV antibodies, were divided into three groups defined by knowledge of their own HIV serostatus: HIV seropositive, HIV seronegative, and those who did not know their serostatus. There were no significant differences in self-reported anal intercourse, number of sexual partners, or condom use among the groups in either sample. Because the study analyzed sexual practices at one point in time following disclosure of HIV serostatus, it is possible that it missed changes in these practices occurring over time.

However, these findings have been replicated among 56 gay and bisexual men by Huggins, Elman, Baker, Forrester, and Lyter (1991). Although the sample as a whole showed a significant decrease in anal intercourse as a passive partner over 6 months, the amount of decrease was not significantly different among the 22 seropositives, 22 seronegatives, and 12 men who did not learn their serostatus.

Fox, Odaka, Brookmeyer, and Polk (1987) tested 1,001 gay and bisexual men for HIV antibodies, of whom 67% elected to receive their results. All of the subjects were counseled to practice safer sex. Analyses were conducted comparing notified HIV-seronegatives, notified HIV-seropositives, and individuals who were not notified of their HIV serostatus. Notified HIV-seropositives showed a greater decrease in the number of sexual partners with whom they had receptive anal intercourse and the number of sexual partners with whom they had insertive anal intercourse than did the not-notified men. In contrast, the notified HIV-seronegatives showed a smaller decrease in total number of sexual partners, number of sexual partners with whom they had receptive anal intercourse, and the number of sexual partners with whom they had insertive anal intercourse than did the not-notified men. This latter result may mean that notification of negative antibody test result implies to individuals that they are in some way "protected" because previous sexual practices did not lead to HIV infection. In this view, awareness of HIV-seronegative status may actually work to increase risk-associated behavior, through creating an illusion of invulnerability. However, the results provide only limited support for this interpretation, inasmuch as the investigators did not demonstrate that the notified seronegative men showed a smaller decrease in risk behavior than did unnotified men who were seronegative specifically.

McCusker et al. (1988) tested 270 asymptomatic gay men for HIV antibodies. Of the 200 men who chose to receive their test results, 151 were seronegative and 49 were seropositive. Of the 70 who chose not to receive their results, 52 were seronegative and 18 were seropositive. All of the men received information about the meaning of the HIV antibody test and HIV risk-reduction strategies. The men completed a questionnaire about their sexual practices prior to HIV antibody testing and at 6-month and 1-year follow-up assessments. There were substantial declines in the number of casual homosexual partners and the number of anogenital partners (insertive and receptive) over the time period, but no effects of serostatus or knowledge of serostatus. A multiple regression analysis on insertive anogenital contact at the 1-year follow-up revealed significant effects of serostatus, awareness of serostatus, and the interaction of serostatus and awareness, controlling for initial behavior. The investigators reported that these effects indicated that seropositives who knew their serostatus showed the greatest decline in risky sexual practices, whereas seropositives who did not know their serostatus showed the smallest decline.

An additional analysis was performed to investigate the change from unprotected to protected anogenital contact or elimination of unprotected anogenital contact. Among men who reported some un-protected anogenital contact at the initial visit, there was a significant interaction between serostatus and knowledge of serostatus. Men who became aware of a positive result were less likely to continue insertive contact without a condom than were seropositive men unaware of their result. Among seronegative men, in contrast, those aware of their result were somewhat *more* likely to continue this practice. This latter finding is consistent with the view that negative test results may not prompt safer behavior change.

A cross-sectional study by Frazer, McCamish, Hay, and North (1988) also found that notification of seronegative status was not associated with increased safer sexual practices. Frazer et al. tested 318 gay and bisexual men for HIV antibodies in Brisbane, Australia. Twenty-three subjects were identified as HIV seropositive, of whom 11 were already aware of their serostatus; 295 tested seronegative, of whom 110 were already aware. Insertive anal intercourse in the previous 6 months was significantly less common among the aware seropositives than among the unaware seropositives. For seronegatives, however, awareness of HIV serostatus was unrelated to frequency of anal intercourse. A separate analysis was done on the 208 subjects who reported anal intercourse at least once within the previous 3 months. The men who had been rested previously were marginally ($p = .06$) more likely to have used a condom during anal intercourse in the previous 3 months than were those who had not been tested. Those who had been tested and were seropositive were significantly more likely always to use a condom when having anal intercourse than were those who previously had been shown to be negative. Condom use did not differ between those who had previously received negative HIV test results and those who had not been tested. Receiving positive results apparently led to less insertive anal intercourse and more condom use, whereas receiving negative results had little impact on either behavior. On the other hand, because no measures were collected prior to testing, the results are difficult to interpret.

Ostrow et al. (1989) collected data from 474 gay men before disclosure of serostatus and about 1 year after. Although there was an overall decrease in sexual behavior, none of the differences between notified and not-notified men within the HIV-seropositive and HIV-seronegative subsamples were statistically significant.

Doll et al. (1990) compared data from 181 gay and bisexual men (51 seropositives and 130 seronegatives) who had elected to learn their HIV results with that from 128 (39 seropositives and 89 seronegatives) who declined to learn their results. These data were also compared to the self-reported behavior of two thirds of these men 3 years earlier. There were significant declines over time in anal intercourse. However, these declines were independent of HIV serostatus, awareness of serostatus, and the interaction of serostatus and awareness of serostatus. Although seropositives had a higher risk index for insertive anal intercourse with casual partners, only 8% of the entire sample had engaged in this very high risk practice in the preceding year. Doll et al. hypothesized that the effects on individuals of learning serostatus might be greatest immediately after disclosure. However, contrary to the hypothesis, there was no relationship between length of time since learning of HIV serostatus and persistence of high-risk behavior.

CONSEQUENCES OF HIV ANTIBODY TESTING

Based on our review, we would offer four tentative conclusions about the effects of HIV antibody testing on psychological distress and HIV risk–associated behavior. First, the studies indicate that people who learned that they were HIV seropositive experienced a transient increase in psychological distress in comparison with HIV-seropositive individuals who chose not to learn their antibody test results. Second, people who learned they were HIV seronegative experienced an immediate reduction in psychological distress that was sustained over time, compared with seronegatives who chose not to learn their antibody test results. Third, people who learned they were HIV seropositive curtailed their HIV risk–associated behavior, compared with seropositives who did not choose to learn their antibody rest results. Fourth, the effects of testing on behavior were less clear for those who received negative results. People who learned they were HIV seronegative did not consistently curtail or increase HIV risk–associated behavior compared with those who chose not to learn their antibody test results.

Mediators

Although there is tentative support for these conclusions, a number of questions must be addressed. For example, although studies generally show that receiving positive test results is associated with a decrease in risky sexual behavior, the causes are unclear and may be multifaceted. Widespread behavior change occurred in many people at risk for AIDS before the availability of HIV antibody testing. This is particularly the case for gay and bisexual men in major cities, the subject population in many of the studies we reviewed (Stall, Coates, & Hoff, 1988; Frazer et al., 1988; Becker & Joseph, 1988). Future studies must distinguish between general behavior change that is influenced by social norms or broad-based community education, as opposed to specific behavior change that results from testing.

Moreover, to design effective interventions, it is necessary to examine the motives behind behavioral reactions to testing. It is possible that the risks of certain practices become more salient after testing positive and this causes a shift to safer behavior. Seropositives may decrease risky behavior because they feel a general social responsibility to protect others or they want to protect a specific partner. Alternatively, seropositives may have fewer opportunities to engage in risky sexual behavior. In one study, 88% of tested individuals planned to tell their primary sexual partners about their HIV serostatus and 78% intended to inform their secondary sexual partners (Kegeles, Catania, & Coates, 1988). Clearly, if partners are told, they may be less willing to engage in risky sexual behavior and may either insist on safer sexual activities or choose to leave the relationship. In fact, there is evidence that seropositives are more likely than are seronegatives to experience the break-up of a relationship (Coates et al., 1987).

Seropositives may also become depressed at their test results and consequently may withdraw socially, reducing their opportunities for sexual involvement. Unfortunately, although studies have measured both psychological distress and reduced risk behavior following HIV-serostatus notification, they have not examined whether effects of seropositive notification on behavior are mediated by psychological distress. Those who receive positive results have also been negatively reinforced for engaging in risky behavior through infection with HIV, which may enhance their motivation for behavior change.

For some seronegatives, increased salience of risks may be a consequence of testing that translates into safer behavior. But the studies did not reveal consistent reductions of risk behavior among seronegatives. Some studies showed increased risk behavior. One possible explanation of this finding is that some seronegative individuals who have previously engaged in high-risk sexual practices receive positive reinforcement when they learn they have not contracted HIV, despite their risky behavior. This may lead to a false sense of protection or invulnerability from HIV infection (Schecter et al., 1988; Kelly & St. Lawrence, 1987). Therefore, receiving negative results may lead to a reduction in the perceived threat of HIV infection and limit motivation to change behavior. Another possibility, however, is that some individuals who test negative may receive little support for behavior change from partners because now partners may perceive they have little reason to fear infection from them.

Selection Bias

Most of the studies examined only individuals who elected to be tested and therefore the samples are self-selected. The results, accordingly, may apply to only a subset of people. Individuals who participate in a study on HIV testing and/or elect to receive their test results may be more or less anxious or depressed about getting AIDS or risk aversive than are those who choose not to participate. Indeed, the fear of possible adverse reactions to receiving positive results is a common barrier to testing among people who engaged in high-risk behavior (Lyter, Valdiserri, Kingsley, Amoroso, & Rinaldo, 1987; Dawson et al., 1991). In one study, 48% of the men who declined to receive results reported that receiving a positive HIV result would be "too worrisome," and 31% expected that they would be "unable to cope" with a positive test result. Thus the effects of providing HIV-seropositive feedback to these individuals might be more deleterious than was observed in the studies we reviewed.

Those who choose to be tested also may have already decided to start to practice safer sex behaviors. For them, getting tested may be part of a broader goal to reduce high-risk behavior and protect their health (Rugg et al., 1991). Although no studies have examined potential differences between individuals who volunteered to be tested and those who did not, studies have examined differences between those who elected to receive their test results and those who did not. In one sample, 40% wanted their results because they believed it would help promote a change in their sexual behavior (Lyter et al., 1987). In another study, those who chose to receive the results of their HIV tests reported greater efforts to change their sexual behavior than did those who were tested and declined notification, although there were no significant differences between these groups on reported behavior (McCusker et al., 1988).

In future studies, it will be important to explore whether certain individuals are at greater risk for adverse reactions in the face of a positive test result (Miller et al., 1992). It is possible, for example, that seropositives who elect to be notified are better able to tolerate the impact of their disease states than are those who shun such testing.

Heterosexual Populations

Ethnic minority members. As shown in Tables 5.1 and 5.2, the majority of studies on the psychological and behavioral consequences of HIV antibody testing have been conducted on white gay and bisexual men. Moreover, the behavioral outcomes of interest have been sexual practices. Although white men who have sex with other men represent the majority of AIDS cases, they are not the only population at risk of HIV infection. Members of ethnic minorities, particularly blacks and Hispanics, are disproportionately represented among people who have AIDS. Blacks and Hispanics compose 20% of the population of the United States, but 43% of reported AIDS cases have involved blacks and Hispanics. In addition, the 1991 National Health Interview Survey indicated that, excluding testing associated with blood donations, the percentage of adults who have been tested for HIV is greater among blacks (22%) and Hispanics (20%) than among whites (12%). Moreover, the percentage expecting to be tested in the next 12 months is also greater among blacks (20%) and Hispanics (11%) than among whites (6%). Blacks and Hispanics were particularly underrepresented in studies of behavioral consequences of testing. Few of these studies included a substantial number of black participants, and none included a substantial number of Hispanics. As a result, little is known about the consequences of testing among ethnic minority groups.

Injection-drug users. Similarly, we know very little about the reactions to HIV antibody testing of injection-drug users. Indeed, none of the studies explored the effects of testing on injection-drug use. Yet over 20% of reported AIDS cases have been tied to injection-drug use, and the percentage is even higher among low-income black and Hispanic individuals. Given that these individuals are faced with a variety of other stresses, the psychological and behavioral consequences of HIV antibody testing might be less dramatic among them than among the more affluent, white middle-class gay men who have been the subjects in the majority of studies.

Measuring Consequences of HIV Testing

Research on changes in HIV risk–associated sexual behavior must rely upon self-reports, which introduces the possibility of self-presentation biases. People who are HIV seropositive are clearly aware that they pose a substantial risk to their sexual partners and of the importance of safer sex practices. One potential consequence of these powerful demand characteristics is that they may report less risky behavior following notification of serostatus, regardless of their actual behavior. Measurement is also complicated because these reports are retrospective, in some studies over substantial time periods. Quite apart from self-representation concerns, individuals may have difficulty recalling accurately their past sexual behavior. Although some research has suggested that self-reports have validity (Catania et al., 1990; Coates et al., 1986; McLaws et al., 1990), there is a need for methods to increase the validity and reliability of self-reports in the context of research on reactions to HIV antibody testing. Some recent studies have trained the interviewers in memory-elicitation techniques, including the use of calendars to prod recall (Rugg et al., 1991).

Researchers might also consider including objective measures as a supplement to self-reports. For example, studies could examine effects of HIV antibody testing on the incidence of sexually transmitted diseases (or, in women, the incidence of pregnancy) rather than relying solely on self-reports of condom use and number of sexual partners. Studies on psychological distress and HIV antibody testing have made some inroads along these lines. Drawing upon research linking psychological stress to neuroendocrine and immunological changes (e.g., Jemmott & Locke, 1984; O'Leary, 1990), studies have used not only self-report measures of psychological distress, but also biological assays of neuroendocrine and immune parameters to gauge reactions to antibody testing (see Antoni, Schneiderman, et al., 1991; and Antoni, Baggett, et al., 1991).

In conclusion, a growing number of people are undergoing HIV antibody testing. The implications of the results of HIV antibody testing for the individual can be profound. Those who are seropositive face the prospect of a stigmatizing and fatal condition. The research reviewed in this chapter suggests that people react with substantial emotional distress, but that they generally cope emotionally with this information within a relatively short period of time. Moreover, HIV-seropositive individuals seem to reduce their HIV risk–associated sexual behaviors. The effects on seronegative men are less clear-cut. The mechanisms that underlie the effects of serostatus notification on behavior are not yet well established. The study populations have been largely limited to white gay men in cities of high rates of infection. Injection-drug users and ethnic minority members, along with issues of needle-use behavior and fertility-related decisions, have received virtually no empirical attention. Although some headway has been made in the area of psychosocial adjustment, considerably more research is needed before the effects of HIV antibody testing on psychopathology and HIV risk–associated behavior can be fully understood.

ACKNOWLEDGMENTS

Preparation of this manuscript was supported in part by grants MH45668 from the National Institute of Mental Health and HD24921 from the National Institute of Mental Health to John B. Jemmott, III; a National Science Foundation Graduate Fellowship to Catherine A. Sanderson; and grants CA 46591 from National Cancer Institute and PBR-71 and PBR-72 from the American Cancer Society to Suzanne M. Miller.

REFERENCES

Antoni, M. H., Baggett, L., Ironson, G., LaPerriere, A., August, S., Klimas, N., Schneiderman, N., & Fletcher, M. (1991). Cognitive-behavioral stress management intervention buffers distress responses and immunologic changes following notification of HIV-1 seropositivity. *Journal of Consulting and Clinical Psychology, 59*(6), 906–915.

Antoni, M. H., Schneiderman, N., Klimas, N., LaPerriere, A., Ironson, G., & Fletcher, M. A. (1991). Disparities in psychological, neuroendocrine, and immunologic patterns in asymptomatic HIV-1 seropositive and seronegative gay men. *Biological Psychiatry, 29,* 1023–1041.

Becker, M. H., & Joseph, J. G. (1988). AIDS and behavior change to reduce risk: A review. *American Journal of Public Health, 78*(4), 394–410.

Blaney, N. T., Millon, C., Morgan, R., Eisdorfer, C., & Szapocznik, J. (1990). Emotional distress, stress-related disruption and coping among healthy HIV-positive gay males. *Psychology and Health, 4,* 259–273.

Catania, J. A., Gibson, D. R., Chitwood, D. D., & Coates, T. J. (1990). Methodological problems in AIDS behavioral research: Influences on measurement error and participation in studies of sexual behavior. *Psychological Bulletin, 108,* 339–362.

Cleary, P. D., Singer, E., Rogers, T. F., Avorn, J., Van Devanter, N., Soumerai, S., Perry, S., & Pindyck, J. (1988). Sociodemographic and behavioral characteristics of HIV antibody–positive blood donors. *American Journal of Public Health, 78*(8), 953–957.

Coates, T. J., Morin, S. F., & McKusick, L. (1987). Behavioral consequences of AIDS antibody testing among gay men. *Journal of the American Medical Association, 258*(14), 1989.

Coates, T. J., Soskolne, C. L., Calzavara, L. M., Read, S. E., Fanning, M. M., Shepard, F. A., Klein, M. M., & Johnson, J. K. (1986). The reliability of sexual histories in AIDS-related research: Evaluation of an interview-administered questionnaire. *Canadian Journal of Public Health, 778,* 343–348.

Coates, T. J., Stall, R. D., Kegeles, S. M., Lo, B., Morin, S. F., & McKusick, L. (1988). AIDS antibody testing: Will it stop the AIDs epidemic? Will it help people infected with HIV? *American Psychologist, 43*(11), 859–864.

Croyle, R. T., & Jemmott, J. B. III. (1991). Psychological reactions to risk factor testing. In J. A. Skelton & R. T. Croyle (Eds.), *The mental representation of health and illness,* (pp. 85–107). New York: Springer-Verlag.

Dawson, J., Fitzpatrick, R., McLean, J., Hart, G., & Boulton, M. (1991). The HIV test and sexual behavior in a sample of homosexually active men. *Social Service and Medicine, 32*(6), 683–688.

Doll, L. S., O'Malley, P. M., Pershing, A. L., Darrow, W. W., Hessol, N. A., & Lifson, A. R. (1990). High-risk sexual behavior and knowledge of HIV antibody status in the San Francisco city clinic cohort. *Health Psychology, 9*(3), 253–265.

Fox, R., Odaka, N. J., Brookmeyer, R., & Polk, B. F. (1987). Effect of HIV antibody disclosure on subsequent sexual activity in homosexual men. *AIDS, 1*(4), 241–246.

Frazer, I. H., McCamish, M., Hay, I., & North, P. (1988). Influence of human immunodeficiency virus antibody testing on sexual behavior in a "high-risk" population from a "low-risk" city. *The Medical Journal of Australia, 149,* 365–368.

Hardy, A. M., & Dawson, D. A. (1990). HIV antibody testing among adults in the United States: Data from 1988 NHIS. *American Journal of Public Health, 80*(5), 586–589.

Huggins, J., Elman, N., Baker, C., Forrester, R. G., & Lyter, D. (1991). Affective and behavioral responses of gay and bisexual men to HIV antibody testing. *Social Work, 36*(1), 61–66.

Institute of Medicine, National Academy of Sciences. (1988). *Confronting AIDS: Update 1988.* Washington, DC: National Academy Press.

Ironson, G., La Perriere, A., Antoni, M., O'Hearn, P., Schneiderman, N., Klimas, N., & Fletcher, M. A. (1990). Changes in immune and psychological measures as a function of anticipation and reaction to news of HIV-1 antibody status. *Psychosomatic Medicine, 52,* 247–270.

Jemmott, J. B. III, Freleicher, J., & Jemmott, L. S. (1992). Perceived risk of infection and attitudes toward risk groups: Determinants of nurses' behavioral intentions regarding AIDS patients. *Research in Nursing and Health, 15*(4), 295–301.

Jemmott, J. B. III, & Locke, S. E, (1984). Psychosocial factors, immunologic mediation, and human susceptibility to infectious diseases: How much do we know? *Psychological Bulletin, 95,* 78–108.

Jemmott, L. S., Jemmott, J. B. III, & Cruz-Collins, M. (1992). Predicting AIDS patient care intentions among nursing students. *Nursing Research, 41,* 172–177.

Kaisch, K., & Anton-Culver, H. (1989). Psychological and social consequences of HIV exposure: Homosexuals in southern California. *Psychology and Health, 3,* 63–75.

Kegeles, S., Catania, J. A., & Coates, T. J. (1988). Intentions to communicate positive HIV-antibody status to sex partners. *Journal of the American Medical Association, 259,* 216–217.

Kelly, J. A., & St. Lawrence, J. S. (1987). *The AIDS health Crisis: Psychological and Social Interventions.* New York: Plenum Press.

Landis, S. E., Earp, J. L., & Koch, G. G. (1992). Impact of HIV testing and counseling on subsequent sexual behavior. *AIDS Education and Prevention, 4*(4), 61–70.

La Perriere, A., Antoni, M. H., Schneiderman, N., Ironson, G., Klimas, N., Caralis, P., & Fletcher, M. A. (1990). Exercise intervention attenuates emotional distress and natural killer cell decrements following notification of positive serologic status for HIV-1. *Biofeedback and self-regulation, 15,* 229–242.

Lyter, D. W., Valdiserri, R. O., Kingsley, L. A., Amoroso, W. P., & Rinaldo, C. R., Jr. (1987). The HIV antibody test: Why gay and bisexual men want or do not want to know their results. *Public Health Reports, 102*(5), 468–474.

Magura, S., Shapiro, J. L., Grossman, J. I., Siddiqi, Q., Lipton, D. S., Amann, K. R., Koger, J., & Gehan, K. (1990). Reactions of methadone patients to HIV antibody testing. *Advances in Alcohol & Substance Abuse, 8*(3/4), 97–111.

McCusker, J., Stoddard, A. M., Mayer, K. H., Zapka, J., Morrison, C., & Staltzman, S. P. (1988). Effects of HIV antibody test knowledge on subsequent sexual behaviors in a cohort of homosexually active men. *American Journal of Public Health, 78*(4), 462–467.

McLaws, M., Oldenburg, B., Ross, M. W., & Cooper, D. A. (1990). Sexual behavior in AIDS-related research: Reliability and validity of recall and diary measures. *Journal of Sex Research, 27,* 265–281.

Miller, S. M., Combs, C., Stoddard, E. (1989). Information, coping, and control in patients undergoing surgery and stressful medical procedures. In A. Steptoe and A. Appels (Eds.), *Stress, Personal Control, and Health* (pp. 107–130). New York: Wiley.

Miller, S. M., Robinson, R., Kruss, L., Caputo, G. C., Hauptman, S., Ift, N., & Buckley, M. (1992). Styles of coping with threat: Implications for adaptation to a severe life stressor. Manuscript under review.

Moss, A. R., Bacchetti, P., Osmond, D., Krampf, W., Chaisson, R. E., Stites, D., Wilber, J., Allain, J. P., & Carlson, J. (1988). Seropositivity for HIV and the development of AIDS or AIDS-related condition: Three-year follow-up of the San Francisco General Hospital cohort. *British Medical Journal, 296,* 745–750.

Moulton, J. M., Stempel, R. R., Bacchetti, P., Temoshok,, L., & Moss, A. R. (1991). Results of a one year longitudinal study of HIV antibody test notification from the San Francisco General Hospital cohort. *Journal of Acquired Immune Deficiency Syndromes, 4*(8), 787–794.

O'Leary, A. (1990). Stress, emotion, and human immune function. *Psychological Bulletin, 108*(3), 363–382.

Ostrow, D. G., Joseph, J. G., Kessler, R., Soucy, J., Tal, M., Eller, M., Chmiel, J., & Phair, J. P. (1989). Disclosure of HIV antibody status: Behavioral and mental health correlates. *AIDs Education and Prevention, 1*(1), 1–11.

Perry, S., Fishman, B., Jacobsberg, L., Young, J., & Frances, A. (1991). Effectiveness of psychoeducational interventions in reducing emotional distress after human immunodeficiency virus antibody testing. *Archives of General Psychiatry, 48,* 143–147.

Perry, S., Jacobsberg, L., Card, C. A. L., Ashman, T., Frances, A., & Fishman, B. (1993). Severity of psychiatric symptoms after HIV testing. *American Journal of Psychiatry, 150*(5), 775–779.

Perry, S., Jacobsberg, L., & Fishman, B. (1990). Suicidal ideation and HIV testing. *Journal of the American Medical Association, 263*(5), 679–682.

Perry, S. W., Jacobsberg, L. B., Fishman, B., Weiler, P. H., Gold, J. W. M., & Frances, A. J. (1990). Psychological responses to serological testing for HIV. *AIDS 4*(2), 145–152.

Rugg, D. L., MacGowan, R. J., Stark, K. A., & Swanson, N. M. (1991). Evaluating the CDC program for HIV counseling and testing. *Public Health Reports, 106*(6), 708–713.

Schecter, M. T., Craib, K. J. P., Willoughby, B., Douglas, B., McLeod, W. A., Maynard, M., Constance, P., & O'Shaughnessy, M. (1988). Patterns of sexual behavior and condom use in a cohort of homosexual men. *American Journal of Public Health, 78*(12), 1535–1538.

Schneider, S. G., Taylor, S. E., Hammen, C., Kemeny, M. E., & Dudley, J. (1991). Factors influencing suicide intent in gay and bisexual suicide ideators: Differing models for men with and without human immunodeficiency virus. *Journal of Personality and Social Psychology, 61,* 776–788.

Singer, E., Rogers, T. F., & Cocoran, M. (1987). The polls—A report on AIDS. *Public Opinion Quarterly, 51,* 580–595.

Stall, R. D., Coates, T. J., & Hoff, C. (1988). Behavioral risk reduction for HIV infection among gay and bisexual men: A review of results from the United States. *American Psychologist, 43*(11), 878–885.

Van Griensven, G. J. P., de Vroome, E. R. M., Tielman, R. A. P., Goudsmit, J., de Wolf, F., van der Noordaa, J., & Coutinho, R. A. (1989). Effect of human immunodeficiency virus (HIV) antibody knowledge on high-risk sexual behavior with steady and nonsteady sexual partners among homosexual men. *American Journal of Epidemiology, 129*(3), 596–603.

Van Griensven, G. J. P., de Vroome, E. M. M., Tielman, R. A. P., Goudsmit, J., Van Der Noordaa, J., De Wolf, F., & Coutinho, R. A. (1988). Impact of HIV antibody testing on changes in sexual behavior among homosexual men in The Netherlands. *American Journal of Public Health, 78*(12), 1575–1577.

Vanichseni, S., Choopanya, K., Des Jarlais, D. C., Plangsringarm, K., Sonchai, W., Carballo, M., Friedmann, P., & Friedman, S. R. (1992). HIV testing and sexual behavior among intravenous drug users in Bangkok, Thailand. *Journal of Acquired Immune Deficiency Syndrome, 5*(11), 119–123.

Watkins, K. E., Metzger, D., Woody, G., & McLellan, A. T. (1993). Determinants of condom use among intravenous drug users. *AIDS, 7*, 719–723.

Wenger, N. S., Greenberg, J. M., Hilborne, L. H., Kusseling, E., Mangotich, M., & Shapiro, M. F. (1992). Effect of HIV antibody testing and AIDS education on communication about HIV risk and sexual behavior. *Annals of Internal Medicine, 117*, 905–911.

Wenger, N. S., Linn, L. S., Epstein, M., & Shapiro, M. F. (1991). Reduction of high-risk behavior among heterosexuals undergoing HIV antibody testing: A randomized clinical trial. *American Journal of Public Health, 81*(12), 1580–1585.

Wiktor, S. Z., Biggar, R. J., Melbye, M., Ebbesen, P., Colclough, G., DiGioia, R., Sanchez, W. C., Grossman, R. J., & Goedert, J. J. (1990). Effect of knowledge of human immunodeficiency virus infection status on sexual activity among homosexual men. *Journal of Acquired Immune Deficiency Syndromes, 3*, 62–68.

Zenilman, J. M., Erikson, B., Fox, R., Reichart, C. A., & Hook, E. W. III. (1992). Effect of HIV posttest counseling on STD incidence. *Journal of the American Medical Association, 267*(6), 843–845.

6

The Psychosocial and Behavioral Impact of Health Risk Appraisals

VICTOR J. STRECHER
MATTHEW W. KREUTER

Health Risk Appraisal (HRA) has been defined as "a procedure for using epidemiological and vital statistics data to provide individuals with projections of their personalized mortality risk and with recommendations for reducing that risk, for the purpose of promoting desirable changes in health behavior" (Schoenbach, Wagner, & Beery, 1987). This definition captures the three essential elements of HRA: assessment, estimation, and education (DeFriese & Fielding, 1990). HRA *assesses* individuals' health status and practices, usually by way of self-administered questionnaires and in some cases biomedical measures. From this information, HRA *estimates* their risk of death or disease from each of several causes and provides personalized *educational messages* that indicate ways they can reduce their risk by changing specific behaviors.

HRA is probably the most widely used health education strategy for promoting individual behavior change (DeFriese & Fielding, 1990; Becker & Janz, 1987). As many as 5 to 15 million Americans have participated in HRA or HRA-like programs in worksites, universities, community wellness programs, health fairs, and health care organizations (Schoenbach, 1987). A recent survey showed that HRA activities now take place at nearly 30% of all worksites (Fielding, 1989). Originally developed as a data gathering mechanism to direct physicians' preventive health care activities (Beery et al., 1986), HRA is now also used to enhance program planning and evaluation, to identify those in need of preventive screening procedures, to help recruit participants into health promotion programs, and to provide information directly to individuals to inform, motivate, and facilitate health-directed behav-

126

ior change (DeFriese & Fielding, 1990; Becker & Janz, 1987; Schoenbach, 1987). A good example of these HRA functions is reported by Kellerman, Felts, and Chenier (1992), who recently found one half of all employees of two shifts of a textile plant enrolling in an HRA/ health screening program. These participants consisted primarily of blue collar employees with significant racial and gender diversity. HRA, therefore, may have significant appeal to sociodemographic groups most in need of health promotion programs.

With its appeal, relative low cost, adaptability, and pervasiveness, HRA would seem—on the surface—to be an important strategy for meeting many of the nation's health objectives. However, reviews of the research literature have found little evidence for HRA's efficacy in changing individual behavior (Schoenbach et al., 1987; Beery et al., 1986; Wagner, Beery, Schoenbach, & Graham, 1982). One explanation for this apparent failure, which we will discuss in detail later in this chapter, has been that HRA does not provide individuals with sufficient or meaningful information about *how to make* the behavior changes it prescribes. HRA collects epidemiological risk factor information about its users, calculates their risk based on population mortality data, and provides feedback to the users identifying their risk factors and the health benefit (usually in years of prolonged life expectancy) they can expect by modifying each risk factor. Implicit in the use of HRA is the belief that provision of *risk information alone* will help people change unhealthy behaviors. But these messages are derived from epidemiological risk calculations, largely—if not entirely— uninformed by behavioral science. As Beery et al. (1986) noted:

> Unlike many behavioral and educational interventions, HRA has not developed out of any particular educational or psychological tradition; it therefore lacks the presumption of efficacy that a close connection with a body of theory and associated empirical evidence would bring (p. 36).

With HRA, no consideration is given to the many psychosocial, physiological, and historical factors that have been demonstrated in multiple theoretical frameworks to mediate individual behavior change. In a 1988 National Health Information Center report (Healthfinder, 1988), 52 different health risk appraisal instruments available in the United States were identified. We requested copies of 23 of these and samples of their feedback. Of the 17 returned, none collected psychosocial data from its users or provided individually tailored behavior change information. This limitation of HRA led Becker and Janz (1987) to conclude that "the provision of typical HRA feedback should not (on a theoretical basis) ordinarily be expected to accomplish much beyond information transmission, belief or attitude change, and the induction of some level of motivation" (p. 547).

HRA VIEWED FROM THE PERSPECTIVE OF THE HEALTH BELIEF MODEL

The Health Belief Model (HBM) is useful in examining why, from a theoretical perspective, the current application of HRA may not have behavioral or even prebehavioral effects on its users. HBM conceptualizes behavior change as a function of perceived threat of a negative health outcome and perceived benefits (minus perceived barriers) of taking a particular course of preventive action. It has been demonstrated to predict a wide variety of health behavior change (Becker, 1974; Janz & Becker, 1984). According to the model, an individual's readiness to engage in a given health behavior is determined by his or her perception of personal *susceptibility* to a specific disease and by perceptions of the *severity* of the consequences of the disease. Combined, perceived susceptibility and severity constitute an individual's *perceived threat* of the disease. Assuming the individual perceives some threat or feels some readiness to change, the benefits of specific health behaviors in terms of reducing the threat are weighed against the costs, or barriers to taking action. A cue to action such as a symptom of illness or a media campaign message may also be necessary to trigger the desired behavior. Demographic, personality, and social

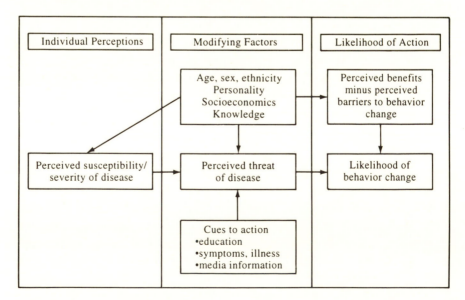

Figure 6.1. Health Belief Model

factors are considered by this model to be modifying factors, affecting behavior only through their influence on other components of the model (Wallston & Wallston, 1984). Figure 6.1 illustrates this model of behavior change.

Viewed from an HBM perspective, typical HRA feedback is found wanting. HRA collects information regarding individuals' health risk factors, including behavioral (e.g., whether you smoke cigarettes, buckle your seat belt, eat excessive amounts of dietary fat), demographic (e.g., your age and gender), and physical status (e.g., your height, weight, blood pressure) variables. These data could be used to develop feedback designed to influence three HBM variables: perceived susceptibility, severity, and the benefits of taking a recommended health-promoting action. But the feedback HRA actually provides to address these variables is limited in content. Typical HRA feedback addresses perceived threat and perceived benefit in purely quantitative terms, usually as the projected number of years of life to

Table 6.1. Health Belief Model (HBM) Concepts Addressed by Typical and Potential Health Risk Appraisal (HRA) Feedback

Health Belief Model Concept	Typical HRA Feedback	Potential HRA Feedback
THREAT		
Perceived susceptibility	Absolute risk estimate for all-cause mortality	Relative risk for specific diseases, injuries, outcomes
Perceived severity	Absolute risk estimate for all-cause mortality	Quantitative and qualitative conceptualization of severity
BENEFIT		
Perceived benefits	Estimated years of life gained by making behavioral changes	Consideration given to quality of life factors
Perceived barriers	None	Identify, address individuals' perceived barriers to change
CUE TO ACTION	HRA may act as a cue to action for individual favorably predisposed to change	Develop behavior specific cues to action
SELF-EFFICACY*	None	Enhance self-efficacy, provide skill-building information to facilitate behavior change

*From Bandura (1977), not HBM; an important related concept some (Rosenstock et al., 1988) suggest should be added to HBM.

be gained or lost by changing or not changing an unhealthy behavior. Yet longevity and being healthy are just two of many factors that might motivate behavior change and arguably not always the most salient ones. Further, because HRA seldom collects data on individuals' motivations for, or concerns about changing their health habits, it has no means of addressing perceived barriers to behavior change, and it does nothing to enhance self-efficacy or build skills necessary to make changes in complex behaviors.

Table 6.1 summarizes HRA's typical treatment of Health Belief Model variables and contrasts it with the kind of feedback that could be provided by HRA if it gathered specific behavior change information and used it to develop individually tailored feedback. The sections following Table 6.1 discuss in greater detail each of the key components of HBM, and how HRA presently does and potentially could address each of them.

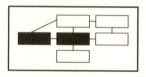

Perceived Susceptibility and Severity, and Perceived Threat

Nearly all information provided in typical HRA feedback is derived from epidemiological risk estimates. HRA usually provides a risk estimate for all-cause mortality (e.g., *"Your 'risk age' is 57.4 years, your actual age is 49.6 years"*), and a breakdown of how specific risk factors contribute to that estimate (e.g., *"If you quit smoking, you can add 4.2 years to your present life expectancy"*). Implicit in the latter message is a kind of threat ("If you continue to smoke, you will cut an average of 4.2 years from your normal life expectancy"). But what are the relative contributions of susceptibility and severity to this threat message? Whether people actually want or need to separate the two concepts in their consideration of risk is unclear (Weinstein, 1988), nor is the relationship made clear in the HBM itself. However, it seems likely that perceptions of risk are made sequentially rather than multiplicatively. For example, a person's perceptions of susceptibility and severity and the resultant *threat* of infection with the AIDS virus versus infection with common cold viruses may radically differ, even though the product of the two perceptions may be similar. The mortality risk estimate feedback provided by HRA does not separate susceptibility from severity. HRA participants may, therefore, receive similar life expectancy decrements from a low-susceptibility/high-severity risk (e.g., HIV transmission) as from a high-susceptibility/low-severity risk (e.g., common cold virus transmission).

In addition, most HRAs convey risk information in terms of *absolute*, rather than relative risk. From an epidemiological standpoint, absolute risk is a less stable measure than is relative risk (Rothman, 1986). From an educational or communication standpoint, it may also be more difficult to understand (Kirscht, 1989). In a study assessing the effects of feedback from four different HRAs on individuals' perceived risk of heart attack, Avis, Smith, & McKinlay (1989) found that the greatest impact on risk perception was achieved by the only HRA of the four that presented risk as relative and specific to a particular outcome (heart attack).

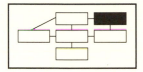

Perceived Benefits Minus Barriers to Behavior Change

Most HRAs provide some feedback regarding the improvement in life expectancy associated with changing a particular behavioral risk factor. But, like HRA's threat messages, these "benefits" are described in purely quantitative terms, usually as the projected years of life to be gained or lost by changing or not changing an unhealthy behavior. To be sure, messages such as "If you were to quit smoking this year, your life expectancy would increase by 4.2 years" may have a positive impact. However, the Health Belief Model emphasizes the user's—not an epidemiologist's—perceived benefits. HRA does not typically ask the user why he or she would like to change a risk factor. If it did, added longevity would not always be a leading response. For example, in an ongoing study of physicians' preventive health care activities (Kreuter, Strecher, & Kegler, 1992), we ask patients expressing interest in making specific health-related behavior changes to give the main reason they wanted to make the change. Among patients interested in exercising more often (n = 141), 40% wanted to do so in order to lose weight, whereas only 22% said they were interested in doing so to improve their health. Granted, losing weight *may* improve their health, for at least 40% of this population, messages focusing on the health benefits of losing weight will probably be less effective than ones emphasizing changes in physical appearance, increased physical capabilities, and self-image that can accompany weight loss. Although some health-related behaviors might be done largely for health reasons, most influential benefits are probably related to a perceived improvement in quality of life (Kaplan, 1985; Kaplan, 1988).

Given HRA's treatment of perceived benefits, the Health Belief Model would predict that recommended changes in health behavior would be attempted only if the user perceived the barriers of engaging in the recommended health action to be quite low. In other words, if a person would like to quit smoking, but perceives stress to be a major barrier to success, HRA alone would not facilitate behavior change. HRA doesn't collect barrier information. This rules out feedback directed toward a broad variety of factors impeding behavior change, from lack of self-efficacy (Bandura, 1977), to physical barriers such as lack of money or time, to lack of knowledge such as where one would go to receive a mammogram. For health behaviors that typically have few barriers, one might expect HRA feedback to be effective. However, for most lifestyle behaviors (e.g., smoking, excessive alcohol use, exercise, diet), HRA feedback would only heighten risk perception. What is the effect of heightening risk perception without addressing the barriers to reducing the risk? People with high risk perception but low efficacy are not likely to change (Strecher, Becker, Kirscht, Eraker, & Graham-Tomasi, 1985). Such a profile, if created, would be an iatrogenic effect of HRA.

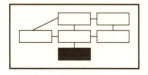

Cues to Action

According to the Health Belief Model, if perceived threat is high and perceived benefits outweigh perceived barriers, a cue to action can prompt or trigger an individual to take a particular health action, in effect stimulating the belief-action link. Cues to action may be internal (e.g., symptoms) or external (e.g., media information). For individuals already highly motivated to change a health behavior, the receipt of HRA feedback confirming their concerns may well serve as an external cue to action (Becker & Janz, 1987). In some cases, however, it seems possible that cues to action may be more effective if they are behavior specific and can be placed in a specific behavioral setting. For example, for relatively simple preventive health practices like wearing seat belts or regularly checking household smoke detectors, a cue to action like a dashboard magnet or calendar sticker would seem to be at least as effective in motivating change as the typical HRA message "If you start buckling your seat belt all the time, you can add 0.1 years to your present life expectancy." HRA could easily provide removable, behavior-specific cues to action as part of its feedback component.

RELATED RESEARCH

To date, research on health risk appraisal has focused primarily on the estimation and education elements of HRA; specifically, the validity of its risk estimates and the effectiveness of its educational feedback. By far, the bulk of published research addresses the former. Although only tangentially related to the proposed study, this line of research bears some mention. In short, there has been considerable debate about the precision of HRA's risk estimation procedures and their ability to predict individuals' future mortality (Wagner et al., 1982). A few recent studies, however, have suggested that some HRAs assess at least certain kinds of risk (e.g., coronary heart disease) fairly accurately (Foxman & Edington, 1987; Smith, McKinlay, & Thorington, 1987). In fact, there seems to be general agreement that although its risk estimates may be imprecise, HRA is sufficiently accurate in distinguishing high from low risk as to justify further testing of its effectiveness as a health promotion tool (Schoenbach, 1987; Wagner et al., 1982; Spasoff & McDowell, 1987; Kannel and McGee, 1987).

The research that does exist on the effectiveness of HRA as strategy for health promotion is, at best, mixed. An early review of HRA effectiveness (Wagner et al., 1982) found the research characterized by methodological weaknesses and only equivocal findings. Among three randomized controlled studies reported, no HRA effect was found on risk factor reduction (Hancock et al., 1978) or attitudes toward disease susceptibility (Cioffi, 1979). The third study (Lauzon, 1977) found small, though inconsistent (across age-sex-risk groups) behavior changes, but was compromised by methodological (attrition, short follow-up) and analytic (unadjusted alpha for multiple outcome analyses) flaws. As of 1987, none of these studies had been published in the scientific literature. Schoenbach and colleagues conducted a similar review in 1987, and again found little convincing evidence in support of HRA. Three new randomized controlled studies were reported on (Smith, Ekdahl, & Henley, 1985; Blue Cross and Blue Shield of Michigan, 1983; Spilman, et al., 1986), one of which (Blue Cross and Blue Shield of Michigan, 1983) was not published in the scientific literature. Among these studies, none provided strong evidence for either psychosocial or behavioral changes resulting from HRA.

A recent study of the impact of HRA and counseling on factory workers found 93% of employees reportedly making a health-related behavior change after receiving HRA and individual counseling from a nurse or health educator (Kellerman et al., 1992). These self-reported changes were in the areas of diet, seat belt use, and cancer screening behaviors (perceptions of risk were not measured). However, a low follow-up rate (57% of those completing both HRA and counseling), lack of an HRA-only group, and lack of a control group limit the inferences that can be made from the results.

Avis and colleagues (1989) conducted a large-scale, well-designed study examining the influence of four HRAs on biases related to perceived heart attack risk. Inaccurate perceptions of risk can be either optimistic or pessimistic. Individuals at high risk who perceive themselves to be at low risk are said to have an optimistic bias; low-risk individuals who perceive themselves to be at high risk, the so-called worried well, have a pessimistic bias. Ideally, HRA should address both types of bias (see Fig. 6.2).

In the Avis study, 732 men and women aged 25 to 65 were randomly selected from the greater Boston area. Subjects received home interviews to determine, among other things, perceived risk of having a

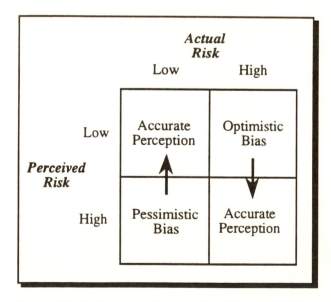

Figure 6.2. Optimistic and Pessimistic Bias in Risk Perception

heart attack within the next 10 years; subjects also received physiological tests of cholesterol, blood pressure, and weight. Upon completion of the interview, subjects were administered one of four randomly assigned HRAs (CDC, Arizona Heart Test, RISKO, and Determine Your Medical Age) or did not receive any HRA. Comparing subjects' perceived risk with an objective measure of their coronary heart disease risk (the risk equation from the Carter Center Healthier People HRA), 42% were found to underestimate their risk, 18% overestimated their risk, and 40% accurately assessed their risk. Subjects were re-interviewed 7 to 12 weeks later.

Of those who initially underestimated their risk (an optimistic bias) who received HRA feedback, 22% increased their perceived risk level, 66% did not change their perceived risk, and 12% decreased their perceived risk. HRA feedback did not influence users with a pessimistic bias. Risk perception among subjects with a pessimistic bias was as likely to increase as it was to decrease after receiving HRA feedback, suggesting there is room for improvement in HRA's treatment of this group.

Research by Weinstein (1982, 1983, 1984) and others (Niknian, McKinlay, Rowowski, & Carleton, 1989; Kulic & Mahler, 1987) suggests that a majority of study subjects may possess optimistic biases regarding their health. Weinstein suggests that optimistic bias is in large part a function of cognitive errors. One error studied by Weinstein is egocentrism—the assumption that other people of similar age, sex, and general situation are not taking the same degree of precautionary action. In a study (Weinstein, 1983) testing the impact of information designed to counteract egocentrism by offering subjects information about the precautionary actions of others, optimistic bias was reduced. An unexpected finding of this study was that subjects in a group instructed to simply describe their own risk factors (with no feedback about others) had the greatest level of optimistic bias. It is possible that consideration of one's own risk factors (or lack of them) actually increases egocentrism and, therefore, optimistic bias.

HRA typically does not provide feedback regarding the health habits of others; rather, its focus is on the individual user and his or her health habits. Based on the Weinstein (1983) study, one wonders whether this focus might actually create unintended egocentrism. HRA users may pay particular attention to risk factors they did not have or ones they had never considered previously. For example, the HRA user may focus on the fact that he always buckles his seat belt and eats lots of vegetables, rather than the fact that he smokes cigarettes. If this is the case, many HRAs may be inviting egocentrism by presenting their mortality risk estimates in terms of absolute rather than relative risk. In other words, although population estimates provide the basis for HRA's risk estimates, most HRAs do not consider this information in the formulation of feedback messages for the user. Interestingly, of the four HRAs administered in the Avis et al. (1989) study, feedback from only one was found to have an effect on perceived risk: the Arizona Heart Institute HRA. This HRA specifically informs people that, compared with others, they are at above average, average, or below average risk for developing heart disease. This would support the hypothesis that optimistic bias is a function of egocentrism, which can, in turn, be counteracted by comparison with others.

Even when HRA does influence risk perception, it may not affect health-related behavior. Avis and colleagues (1989) found no evidence that changes in risk perception led to behavior changes to decrease heart attack risk (e.g., smoking, exercise, dietary control). This is not surprising. According to the Health Belief Model, we would not necessarily expect behavior change to have occurred. Only in cases where the behavior is relatively free of significant psychological and physical barriers (e.g., wearing seat belts) would be expected changes in risk perception to affect changes in behavior.

Although no study could be found that examined the relationship between perceived barriers and HRA impact, unpublished research by Sloan and Gemson (1991) examines the role of motivation on HRA impact. In a randomized trial of a computerized version of the Centers for Disease Control HRA, 161 employees were given a periodic health examination, laboratory tests, and counseling on the basis of this evaluation. These subjects also completed the HRA and were randomly assigned to either receive or not receive the HRA feedback. Six months later, positive physical and lifestyle changes, including improvements in serum cholesterol, weight, physical activity, and seat belt usage as well as overall improvement (lowering) of HRA appraised age were found among subjects who had a higher HRA-appraised age than their actual chronological age (what the authors termed the "high motivation" group) and who received the HRA feedback. Like the Kellerman et al. study, this trial had a low rate of follow-up (57%). However, they did have the advantage of a comparison group not receiving HRA feedback.

It is possible to interpret the Sloan and Gemson results in several ways. The behavior changes made by these "highly motivated" subjects could have been considered relatively simple, with few perceived barriers (though the weight reduction results found in this study appear to work against this argument). Or, the health counseling administered to both groups may have had a greater impact on the group receiving the HRA. Not knowing what was administered in these counseling sessions limits the evidence for or against this possibility. Finally, it is possible that strong motivation supersedes barriers to change. Support for this argument (which would appear to run contrary to our assertion that barriers should be addressed by HRA) also comes from research by Jackson, Stapleton, Russell, and Merriman (1986), who found that smokers with high motivation to quit had high success rates regardless of number of cigarettes smoked at baseline (an indication of nicotine dependency), whereas smokers with lower levels of motivation were strongly influenced by baseline cigarette consumption.

Dunton, Perkins, and Zopf (1990) examined the influence of HRA on seat belt use in six worksite settings. Worksites were assigned to one of three conditions: HRA and a group counseling session, HRA and group counseling plus educational materials designed to facilitate habit change, or a control condition. Seat belt use would appear to be a relatively simple behavior influenced more by outcome expectations than by efficacy expectations (Strecher, DeVellis, Becker, & Rosenstock, 1986). Because the barriers to seat belt use are relatively minimal, we would expect HRA, on the basis of the Health Belief Model, to have a greater impact on this practice. We would also expect the use of behavior change strategies to be unnecessary.

In the Dunton et al. study, seat belt use was observed at each worksite at baseline, after screening, after counseling, and 2 to 3 months later. Worksites with the HRA plus group counseling program showed a greater increase in seat belt use over the course of the study than did the control worksites. Worksites receiving the HRA plus educational materials actually showed smaller increases in seat belt use than did HRA plus group counseling worksites. Although these results suggest that HRA may be able to influence simple health behaviors like seat belt use, it is important to recognize at least two of its limitations. First, the study did not test a true HRA-only condition; all HRA feedback was supplemented with group counseling. Second, the study did not assess subjects' baseline perceived risk and thus does not establish a link between HRA-induced risk perception or awareness and the behavior of seat belt use.

Because no HRA currently assesses psychosocial factors and provides tailored behavior change feedback, the efficacy of such treatment cannot be directly assessed. However, preliminary data from our own research study suggest that existing HRAs may not be addressing users' behavior change needs and interests in an optimal way. In a vanguard trial, 541 patients from four community medical practices in North Carolina completed a questionnaire identifying their risky behaviors (Kreuter et al., 1992). For the behaviors they were interested in changing, it also assessed appropriate related psychosocial factors. For example, patients were asked to identify the main reason they wanted to make a particular change. If typical HRA feedback addresses perceived benefits at all, it does so only in terms of health and life longevity outcomes. Yet, as we have mentioned, our data indicate that those are by no means the only factors motivating lifestyle change, and in many cases not even the most important ones. Further, the factors motivating change vary from one behavior to the next and include reasons as diverse as "friends and family members want me to," "to relieve stress," "because it's the law," and "to save money." A more theoretically based HRA would identify these factors and tailor individual feedback messages appropriately. Data from our vanguard trial (Table 6.2), shows patients' "main reasons" for wanting to make changes in six specific health-related behaviors.

In our vanguard trial, patients were also asked to identify factors that would keep them from making the changes they had expressed interest in (barriers). Patients identified as many barriers as they perceived to be important to them. Data on patients' perceived barriers are presented in Table 6.3. Given the complex nature of many of these barriers (e.g., stress, lack of time, lack of social support), it seems highly unlikely that typical HRA feedback could be effective in helping users change a broad range of health-related behaviors. Note, however, that the most common barrier to seat belt use is forgetfulness. This is

Table 6.2. Patients' Main Reasons for Wanting to Make Changes in Health-Related Behaviors

Main Reasons for Wanting to. . .	Most Common Response (%)	2nd Most Common Response (%)	3rd Most Common Response (%)
exercise more often (n=254)	control my weight (39.8)	improve my health (22.0)	relieve stress (15.4)
drink less alcohol (n=46)	improve my health (37.0)	feel better about myself (26.1)	take control of my life (17.4)
eat less fat (n=282)	control my weight (48.9)	improve my health (31.2)	feel better (9.6)
quit smoking (n=98)	improve my health (56.1)	friends, family want me to (8.2)	to save money (7.1)
wear seat belts (n=34)	to prevent injuries (47.1)	to feel safer (17.6)	because it's the law (14.7)

Source: Kreuter et al., 1992.

Table 6.3. Patients' Perceived Barriers to Changing Specific Health-Related Behaviors

Main Barriers to...	Most Common Response (%)	2nd Most Common Response (%)	3rd Most Common Response (%)
exercising more often (n=254)	no time (63.7)	don't want to exercise alone (16.9)	bored with exercise (14.2)
drinking less alcohol (n=46)	enjoy drinking (41.3)	helps me relax (21.7)	my friends drink (19.6)
eating less fat (n=282)	like taste of high-fat foods (45.7)	preparing low-fat foods is too difficult (10.6)	friends and/or family don't want to (10.6)
quitting smoking (n=98)	stress (68.4)	low self-efficacy (23.5)	weight gain (22.4)
wearing seat belts (n=34)	forget to use (85.3)	comfort (20.6)	fear of injury (11.8)

Source: Kreuter et al., 1992.

a comparatively minor barrier and may be amenable to change by risk information alone or by a simple reminder, or "cue to action."

Our preliminary research has demonstrated the ability to identify these and other psychosocial variables and to create individually tailored behavior change messages designed to address them. The apparent feasibility of this approach makes it promising for application to HRA, particularly if such messages are shown to have a positive effect on factors influencing behavior or upon behavior itself.

RECOMMENDATIONS

Considering the popularity and continuing dissemination of HRA in worksite and medically based health promotion programs, careful attention to potential improvements of HRA seem warranted. From our analysis of the psychosocial and behavioral effects of HRA, we can make a number of recommendations for changes and for further research.

1. *Provide feedback that allows the user to understand his or her risk status relative to others in the population.* As discussed previously in this chapter, most HRAs use behavioral and nonbehavioral information to provide an actual mortality estimate. Using population-based data to create individualized feedback is not scientifically justifiable and probably not effective in changing risk perceptions or behavior. We recommend simple feedback similar to the question of perceived risk asked by Weinstein in his research: "your risk of dying prematurely from

(disease x) is (greater/about the same/less than) the risk of other (men/women) of your age." A corollary to this recommendation is to provide stronger positive feedback for users with a pessimistic bias. Individuals who have good health habits and are at low risk should be told so.

2. *Provide feedback that allows the user to better understand the relative risks of diseases he or she is at risk of acquiring.* Voluntary health agencies and federal health institutions tend to identify categorical health problems and inform the public of the dangers of those problems. Almost never do these organizations inform the public of the relative risks of acquiring one disease versus acquiring other diseases. For example, the public often hears about the increasing risk of acquiring melanoma (a malignant skin cancer), though almost nothing is mentioned of the risk of acquiring skin cancer (which has an absolute lifetime risk of about 1 in 100) versus the risk of other, more prevalent, cancers such as breast cancer (which has an absolute lifetime risk among women of about 1 in 10).

3. *Provide feedback that allows the user to better understand the relative impact of various risk factors.* Although the public can cite major health risk factors, they often are inaccurate in their rankings of the magnitude of these factors. Many people, for example, view smoking and high cholesterol as cardiovascular disease risk factors of similar magnitude. However, the cardiovascular risk from smoking, for most people, far exceeds the cardiovascular risk of eating foods high in cholesterol or saturated fat. HRA should be an appropriate mechanism for clearly presenting the relative impact of various risk factors, including behavioral (e.g., smoking, diet, seat belt use) and nonbehavioral (e.g., family history, age, gender) factors.

4. *Provide feedback that allows the user to understand the health benefits of specific behavioral changes.* Even though most users of HRA will probably be familiar with the health risks posed by particular behavioral and nonbehavioral factors, many will not have a clear understanding of the benefits derived from changing a targeted behavior. Altering some health-related behaviors has little or no effect on life expectancy among users who belong to certain age groups or who have certain medical conditions. Overstating the effects of health behavior change will have long-term deleterious effects on the credibility of health promotion efforts. On the other hand, some risk factor change effects (e.g., the effects of quitting smoking on existing cardiovascular disease) physical health status in profound and immediate ways.

5. *Provide feedback that enhances the user's ability to make recommended health behavior changes.* As discussed previously, the utility of HRA in changing behavior is currently limited by the characteristics of the behavior in question. Just as HRA currently collects information about health risk and develops feedback tailored to the user, additional components could collect information regarding characteristics of the targeted behavior and develop behavior change messages tailored specifically to these characteristics. We are currently conducting research in the University of North Carolina's Health Communications Research Laboratory that examines whether the assessment of motivation to change, barriers, and other characteristics of the behavior, with subsequent computer-tailored behavior change information, influences the change process over and above traditional HRA feedback. This research primarily uses the stage-based model of change developed by Prochaska and DiClemente (1983) and the Health Belief Model (Becker, 1974; Janz & Becker, 1984) as theoretical frameworks for determining constructs to assess and intervene upon. Future applied research should examine other models of health behavior change in generating HRA assessment factors and in developing the content of personalized feedback.

REFERENCES

Avis, N. E., Smith, K. W., & McKinlay, J. B. (1989). Accuracy of perceptions of heart attack risk: What influences perceptions and can they be changed? *American Journal of Public Health, 79*(12), 1608–1612.

Bandura, A. (1977). Toward a unifying theory of behavior change. *Psychological Review, 84*(2), 191–215.

Becker, M. H. (Ed.). (1974). The health belief model and personal health behavior. *Health Education Monographs, 2*, 324–473.

Becker, M. H., & Janz, N. K. (1987). On the effectiveness and utility of health hazard/health risk appraisal in clinical and nonclinical settings. *Health Services Research*, 537–551.

Beery, W. L., Schoenbach, V. J., Wagner, E. H., et al. (1986). *Health risk appraisal: Methods and programs with annotated bibliography.* (Department of Health and Human Services Publication No. [PHS] 86-3396). Washington, DC: National Center for Health Services Research and Health Care Technology.

Blue Cross and Blue Shield of Michigan. (1983). *Go to Health.* Final report submitted to the Health Services Foundation, Detroit, MI.

Cioffi, J. P. (1979). The effect of health status feedback on health beliefs: An inquiry into the prebehavioral outcomes of a health hazard appraisal. Proceedings of the 15th Annual Meeting on Prospective Medicine and Health Hazard Appraisal. Bethesda, MD: *Health and Education Resources*, 41–47.

DeFriese, G. H., & Fielding, J. E. (1990). Health risk appraisal in the 1990s: Opportunities, challenges, and expectations. *Annual Review of Public Health, 11,* 401–418.

Dunton, S., Perkins, D. D., & Zopf, K. J. (1990). The impact of worksite-based health risk appraisal programs on observed safety belt use. *Health Education Research, 5*(2), 207–216.

Fielding, J. E. (1989). Frequency of health risk assessment activities at U.S. worksites. *American Journal of Preventive Medicine, 5,* 73–81.

Foxman, B., & Edington, D. W. (1987). The accuracy of health risk appraisal in predicting mortality. *American Journal of Public Health, 77*(8), 971–974.

Hancock, J. R., Lees, R. E. M., Binhammer, H. E., et al. (1978). *Patient compliance with health hazard appraisal recommendations.* Kingston, Ontario: Queen's University, Department of Community Health and Epidemiology.

Healthfinder. (1988, November) National Health Information Center, Office of Disease Prevention and Health Promotion, Department of Health and Human Services, Washington, DC.

Jackson, P. H., Stapleton, J. A., Russell, M. A., & Merriman, R. J. (1986). Predictors of outcome in a general practitioner intervention against smoking. *Preventive Medicine, 15*(3), 244–253.

Janz, N. K., & Becker, M. H. (1984). The health belief model: a decade later. *Health Education Quarterly 1984, 11*(1), 1–47.

Kannel, W. B., & McGee, D. L. (1987). Composite scoring—methods and predictive validity: Insights from the Framingham study. *Health Services Research,* 499–535.

Kaplan, R. M. (1985). Quantification of health outcomes for policy studies in behavioral epidemiology. In R. M. Kaplan & M. H. Criqui (Eds.), *Behavioral epidemiology and disease prevention* (pp. 31–54). New York: Plenum.

———. (1988). Health-related quality of life in cardiovascular disease. *Journal of Consulting and Clinical Psychology, 56*(3), 382–392.

Kellerman, S. T., Felts, W. M., Chenier, T. C. (1992). The impact on factory workers of health risk appraisal and counseling in health promotion. *American Journal of Preventive Medicine,* 37–42.

Kirscht, J. P. (1989). Process and measurement issues in health risk appraisal [Editorial]. *American Journal of Public Health, 79*(12), 1598–1599.

Kreuter, M. W., Strecher, V. J., & Kegler, M. C. (1992). *Facilitating preventive care activities in a primary care setting.* Paper presented at the American Public Health Association Meetings, Washington, DC.

Kulik, J. A., & Mahler, H. I. M. (1987). Health status, perceptions of risk and prevention interest for health and non-health problems. *Health Psychology, 6,* 15–27.

Lauzon, R. R. J. (1977, September). *A randomized controlled trial on the ability of health hazard appraisal to stimulate appropriate risk reduction behavior.* Doctoral dissertation, University of Oregon.

Niknian, M., McKinlay, S. M., Rawowski, W., & Carleton, R. (1989). A comparison of perceived and objective CVD risk in a general population. *American Journal of Public Health, 79*(12), 1653–1654.

Prochaska, J. O., & DiClemente, C. C. (1983). Stages and processes of self-change or smoking: Toward an integrative mode of change. *Journal of Consulting and Clinical Psychology, 51,* 390–395.

Rosenstock, I. M., Strecher, V. J., & Becker, M. H. (1988). Social learning theory and the health belief model. *Health Education Quarterly 1988, 15*(2), 175–183.

Rothman, K. J. (1986). *Modern epidemiology* (p. 37). Boston: Little, Brown and Company.

Schoenbach, V. J. (1987). Appraising health risk appraisal [Editorial]. *American Journal of Public Health, 77,* 409–411.

Schoenbach, V. J., Wagner, E. H., & Beery, W. L. (1987). Health risk appraisal: Review of evidence for effectiveness. *Health Services Research,* 553–580.

Sloan, R. P., & Gemson, D. H. (1991, March). *Health risk appraisal, motivation, and behavior change at the worksite.* Paper presented at the Society for Behavioral Medicine meetings, Washington, DC.

Smith, K. W., McKinlay, S. M., & Thorington, B. D. (1987). The validity of health risk appraisal instruments for assessing coronary heart disease risk. *American Journal of Public Health, 77*(4), 419–424.

Smith, W. A., Ekdahl, S. S., & Henley, C. E. (1985). Use of health hazard appraisal in counseling for reduction of risk factors. *Journal of the American Osteopathic Association, 85*(12), 809–814.

Spasoff, R. A., & McDowell, I. W. (1987). Potential and limitations of data and methods in health risk appraisal: risk factor selection and measurement. *Health Services Research,* 467–497.

Spilman, M. A., et al. (1986). Effects of a corporate health promotion program. *Journal of Occupational Medicine, 28*(4), 285–289.

Strecher, V. J., Becker, M. H., Kirscht, J. P., Eraker, S. A., & Graham-Tomasi, R. P. (1985). Psychological aspects of changes in cigarette smoking behavior. *Patient Education and Counseling, 7,* 249–262.

Strecher, V. J., DeVellis, B. M., Becker, M. H., & Rosenstock, I. M. (1986). The role of self efficacy in achieving health behavior change. *Health Education Quarterly 1986, 13*(1), 73–92.

Wagner, E. H., Beery, W. L., Schoenbach, V. J., & Graham, R. M. (1982). An assessment of health hazard/health risk appraisal. *American Journal of Public Health, 72*(4), 347–352.

Wallston, B. S., & Wallston, K. A. (1984). Social psychological models of health behavior: An examination and integration. In A. Baum & J. Singer (Eds.), *Handbook of psychology and health. Vol. IV: Social aspects of health* (pp. 23–53). Hillsdale, NJ: Lawrence Erlbaum.

Weinstein, N. D. (1982). Unrealistic optimism about susceptibility to health problems. *Journal of Behavioral Medicine, 5,* 441–460.

———. (1983). Reducing unrealistic optimism about illness susceptibility. *Health Psychology, 2,* 11–20.

———. (1984). Why it won't happen to me: Perceptions of risk factors and illness susceptibility. *Health Psychology, 3,* 431–457.

———. (1988). The precaution adoption process. *Health Psychology, 7,* 355–386.

7

Understanding the Impact of Risk Factor Test Results: Insights from a Basic Research Program

PETER H. DITTO
ROBERT T. CROYLE

As part of an optional "wellness" program offered by his company, John makes an appointment to take a battery of medical screening tests. John feels well and has no obvious physical complaints. John arrives for his appointment at a medical building, completes a brief health history questionnaire, and has his blood pressure taken. John is then told about a condition called hypercholesterolemia, a high level of cholesterol in the blood, which is a risk factor for cardiovascular disease. John is administered a blood cholesterol test—his finger is pricked and he waits the few minutes to get his total cholesterol count. John is surprised when he is told that his cholesterol level is high (245 mg/dl).

As part of an extra-credit option in her introductory psychology course at college, Jane makes an appointment to serve as a subject in a research project on the health characteristics of college students. Jane feels well and has no obvious physical complaints. Jane arrives for her appointment at the research wing of the psychology department, completes a brief health history questionnaire, and has her blood pressure taken. Jane is then told about a condition called thioamine acetylase (TAA) enzyme deficiency, a risk factor for a complex of mild but irritating pancreatic disorders. Jane is told how to self-administer a test for the presence of TAA—she dips a chemically coated test strip in a sample of her saliva and is told that if the test strip changes color it indicates that she has TAA deficiency. Jane is surprised when her test strip changes from its original yellow color to a dark green.

There are several salient differences between the two scenarios described above. The scenarios differ in the physical context within which the medical test is given, the specifics of how the test is administered, the age and gender of the individuals receiving the diagnostic information, and the familiarity and seriousness of the diagnosed risk factor and its ultimate medical consequences. And yet, it is easy to imagine that John and Jane might have quite similar reactions to the risk factor information each received in their respective scenarios. In fact, it will be our contention in this chapter that these two scenarios are, at least at the level of the psychological reactions expected from the two individuals, very similar. This is important because the central way that the two scenarios differ is that the first describes an actual risk factor screening situation, whereas the second describes one of our laboratory experiments. To the extent that the latter situation is a reasonable psychological analogue of the former, the cognitive, motivational, and social determinants of reactions to actual risk factor information become subject to careful examination in a highly controlled laboratory environment.

In this chapter, we begin by discussing limitations of research on the impact of risk factor testing in public health settings. We then provide a detailed description of our procedure for studying cognitive appraisals of risk factor information in the laboratory and describe the major findings generated by a series of studies using this procedure. In these studies, participants are randomized to different test result conditions. We will focus in particular on the two most commonly observed phenomena in our experimental studies: the denial of the threat represented by an unfavorable test result and the use of social comparison information to evaluate the seriousness and behavioral implications of the health threat. Next, we will examine the generalizability of the experimental findings. The data will show that the results from our basic experimental paradigm are readily replicated when tests are conducted in more realistic contexts, when tests for actual risk factors are used, and when the effects of several well-known individual difference variables are controlled.

Finally, the last part of this chapter will discuss another issue related to generalization: the relationship between cognitive appraisals (the dependent variable in most of our experiments) and health-related behavior (usually the focus of risk factor screening programs). We will discuss a consistent finding in our research that has both theoretical and practical importance: defensive cognitive appraisals and prob-lem-focused coping behavior are functionally independent. If defen-sively optimistic assessments of the threat represented by a risk factor do not necessarily interfere with adaptive coping behavior, then at-tempts to "correct" these assessments may be misguided and, ulti-mately, counterproductive.

LIMITATIONS OF PREVIOUS RISK FACTOR LABELING RESEARCH

The other chapters in this volume review the public health research literature concerning labeling effects. As noted by the other contribu-tors, interpreting this scattered body of work is a difficult task. Not only is the amount of research limited, it is also characterized by a number of methodological limitations. One of the most critical limita-tions is that most of the studies utilize designs that do not test cause-and-effect relationships. The vast majority of studies rely on observa-tional designs that greatly limit the ability of investigators to identify causal links between risk notification and psychosocial responses. Most of the prospective studies do not include control groups. Because risk status is often correlated with many other variables, the effect of communicating different test results is heavily confounded. The only way to eliminate confounds is to randomly assign study participants to different types of test feedback. Therefore, only an experiment that utilizes some form of deception can provide a pure examination of the effects of risk factor test results and the psychological processes underlying these effects.

Although the use of temporary deception in basic psychological research is unfamiliar to many public health researchers, deception has long been used by social psychologists to investigate issues such as conformity, impression formation, persuasion, group conflict, preju-dice, and aggression (Aronson, Ellsworth, Carlsmith, & Gonzales, 1990). One reason why deception is used so often in this research is that social behavior is highly reactive. It is also subject to social desirability motives. For example, research subjects are often unwilling to admit to possessing racist attitudes and beliefs. Therefore, it is not surprising that when Silverman (1974) asked college students to pick a hypotheti-cal roommate, the race of the potential roommate had no influence on selections. On the other hand, when subjects were told that their decision would determine their actual roommate (a deception), race became a significant determinant of selections. This illustrates another reason why deception is used: judgments and behaviors are often substantially different when individuals are highly involved in a situation that has direct personal relevance.

THE FEASIBILITY OF AN EXPERIMENTAL APPROACH TO STUDYING RISK FACTOR TESTING

The psychological dynamics of risk factor screening differ in some important ways from diagnosis in traditional primary care. Primary care patients are often motivated to seek care because of their physical symptoms. They expect and desire a diagnosis, prognosis, and treatment. In these settings, diagnoses are often communicated to individuals who already perceive themselves as ill.

In the case of risk factor screening, many of the individuals who are confronted with risk information are asymptomatic. The central goal in studying labeling effects, therefore, is to achieve an understanding of the psychological effects of *subjective health status*—for example, the belief that one has an elevated risk for a life-threatening disease. By randomizing study participants to different risk information conditions, perceived risk status can be studied in a highly controlled manner. Because risk factor information is typically communicated to individuals who are asymptomatic, healthy populations can be used as subjects.

The TAA Enzyme Paradigm

Spurred on by the belief that risk factor labeling could be studied experimentally in the laboratory, our first step was to develop a viable laboratory analogue of the risk factor testing situation. In collaboration with John Jemmott, we developed a procedure that was intended to recreate the psychological experience of an actual risk factor screening situation while remaining sensitive to the ethical constraints required by an experimental approach. In addition, the procedure was intended to be flexible. Flexibility was important because we hoped to model many different real-world settings, manipulate a wide range of independent variables, and measure many different dependent variables, all while using a standard set of procedures.

The core of the procedure involves bringing study participants into the laboratory and "testing" them for the presence of a fictitious risk factor. Two aspects of the procedure rely on deception. Participants are told that the risk factor is real. In addition, participants are randomly assigned to receive either a positive or a negative test result. Why use a fictitious risk factor? We had four primary reasons. First, the use of a fictitious risk factor controls for individual differences in knowledge and experience. This source of variance has been one of the primary barriers to progress in research on labeling effects. Second, the use of a fictitious risk factor allows for more effective debriefing in that subjects can be told not only that they do not have the risk factor but that the risk factor itself does not exist. Third, the perceived seriousness of a fictitious risk factor can be controlled and consequently set at a level that is minimally sufficient to produce the desired impact. Finally, the use of a fictitious risk factor provides a great deal of experimental flexibility; the investigator is free to control and test the impact of a wide variety of independent variables without contradicting prior knowledge.

So far, all of the studies that have used the enzyme test procedure have employed college students as subjects. Participants are recruited for a study of college students' health characteristics. When students arrive for their appointment, they are met by an experimenter in a white laboratory coat and seated in a room filled with medical paraphernalia (e.g., posters, pamphlets, charts). Participants generally begin the session by completing a health history and having their blood pressure taken. With this context created, subjects are told about a diagnostic test for a condition called "Thioamine Acetylase (TAA) Deficiency." TAA deficiency is said to be a recently discovered enzyme condition that is a risk factor for a complex of "mild but irritating pancreatic disorders."

Participants are told that there is a simple diagnostic test for TAA deficiency that involves dipping a chemically coated test strip in a saliva sample and looking for a color reaction. Participants then self-administer the test. They begin by rinsing their mouths with mouth-wash (ostensibly to cleanse their mouths for the test). The student then places a saliva sample in a cup and "tests" this saliva by immersing a "TAA test strip." This test strip is actually a common urinary glucose test strip. Because a small amount of dextrose has been dissolved in the mouthwash, the test strip turns from yellow to green when placed in contact with the saliva. All participants see this color reaction but are led to interpret it in different ways. The meaning of the test result is manipulated by telling some subjects that the color reaction indicates a positive test result (i.e., TAA deficiency) and telling others that it indicates a negative test result (i.e., normal TAA presence).

After receiving their test result, subjects complete a series of questionnaires in which questions about the fictitious condition and diagnostic test are embedded in similar questions about actual health disorders and diagnostic tests. Medical conditions that are likely to be as unfamiliar as TAA deficiency are included to mask our particular interest in judgments about TAA deficiency. Completion of these questionnaires typically takes less than 10 minutes, after which subjects are thoroughly debriefed.

Reports of subjects after participation suggest that the procedure is quite convincing without causing emotional upset. Although the paradigm relies on deception, suspicion rates are typically very low (5% or less). Subjects perceive TAA deficiency to be about as serious as laryngitis (Ditto, Jemmott, & Darley, 1988). The time between the diagnostic feedback and debriefing is kept at a minimum. Subjects high in hypochondriacal tendencies are often excluded from participation, as are diabetics and hypoglycemics (because of the use of dextrose in the procedure). For further discussion of the paradigm and its limitations, see Croyle and Ditto (1990).

Motivational and Social Determinants of Risk Factor Appraisal: An Initial Investigation

In the first experiment to utilize this procedure, Jemmott, Ditto, and Croyle (1986) provided initial evidence for two phenomena that have become the focus of much of our subsequent research. The first issue addressed by this experiment was whether this procedure could be used to uncover evidence of denial reactions in response to unfavorable medical information. Although denial and other forms of defensiveness in response to illness are well accepted clinically (Hackett & Casem, 1969; Janis, 1958; Kubler-Ross, 1969; Lipowski, 1970), our review of the literature turned up only scattered and indirect empirical evidence of these phenomena. In fact, the very existence of such motivated biases in judgment have been a controversial issue in experimental psychology for over 40 years (Erdelyi, 1974; Miller & Ross, 1975; Tetlock & Levi, 1982). The TAA enzyme procedure is quite useful in exploring evidence of denial in that it isolates the independent variable of interest (level of threat) and allows a direct analysis of causal relationships.

The second issue of interest in the Jemmott et al. study was the role of prevalence information in reactions to risk factor information. Zola (1966) observed that ailments are less likely to stimulate a treatment-seeking response in populations where those ailments are relatively widespread. One interpretation of this finding is that people perceive health disorders as less serious to the extent that they appear to be common. Again, the TAA enzyme procedure seemed perfectly suited to examine this question. By providing participants with different information about the prevalence of TAA deficiency, we could examine the effects of this variable on seriousness judgments.

Jemmott et al. designed an experiment to examine these two issues. Half of the subjects were led to believe they tested positive for TAA deficiency, and half that they tested negative. In addition, half of the subjects were led to believe TAA deficiency was relatively common, and half that it was relatively rare. One obvious way we might have manipulated perceived prevalence was with statistical information. However, we wanted to manipulate prevalence information in a way that more closely resembled how such information is obtained in everyday life. Subjects participated in groups of two or three with each individual in a separate room, but all subjects were led to believe that five subjects were participating in the session. Each subject self-administered the enzyme test and reported the results to the experimenter. In the high-prevalence conditions, the experimenter then told the subject that four of the five students had tested positive for the deficiency. In the low-prevalence conditions, the subject was told that just one of the five students had the deficiency. In this way, the perceived prevalence of TAA deficiency was manipulated by altering its prevalence in the subject's immediate social comparison group.

The results of the study provided strong evidence for both of the predicted effects. Two common forms of denial described in medical patients are minimization of the seriousness of the health threat (Janis, 1958; Lazarus, 1983; Lipowski, 1970) and heightened skepticism regarding the validity of the diagnosis (Visotsky, Hamburn, Goss, & Lebovitz, 1961). After the diagnostic feedback, subjects rated the seriousness of TAA deficiency on a 100-point scale (where 0=not serious, can be ignored and 100-very serious, life-threatening), and the accuracy of the diagnostic test for TAA on a 9-point scale (where 9-very accurate). Subjects who tested positive for TAA deficiency rated it as a significantly less serious threat to health than did subjects who tested negative. Similarly, positive-result subjects rated the saliva reaction test as a significantly less accurate indicator of TAA deficiency than did negative-result subjects. That this effect is due to denial is further supported by the finding that the tendency to denigrate the accuracy of the test was particularly pronounced when subjects believed that they alone had received the positive test result.

The effects of the prevalence manipulation also confirmed our expectations. When subjects believed that only one of the five students had tested positive for TAA deficiency, they perceived the deficiency as significantly more serious than when they believed four of the five students had tested positive. Thus, even though the medically significant information about the deficiency was exactly the same in both conditions, subjects rated the enzyme condition as more serious when it appeared to be rare than when it appeared to be common.

The Jemmott et al. experiment provided support for the viability of an experimental approach to studying risk factor appraisals as well as evidence of two important determinants of such appraisals. Subsequent research has expanded on both of the major findings of this study, and each of these lines of research will be discussed in turn.

DENIAL OF RISK FACTOR INFORMATION

Are the relatively optimistic threat appraisals of positive-result subjects the project of a defensive motivational process like denial or of some more rational aspect of information processing? Given our desire to understand the labeling process, one focus of our subsequent research with the TAA paradigm has been to rule out competing, nonmotivational explanations for the effect of favorability of test results on threat-related appraisals. Not only has this work confirmed the motivational nature of this phenomenon, but, along the way, many interesting findings have emerged regarding the conditions under which denial reactions are most likely to be observed and the wide variety of forms such denial reactions are likely to take.

Denial and Confirmatory Symptom Reporting

One alternative explanation for the denial effects observed in the Jemmott et al. study hinges on the differential symptom information that was potentially available to positive and negative test result subjects. Healthy college students who are told that they have an abnormal health condition may have special knowledge about it—that people (like themselves) who have the disorder do not feel ill. In other words, if we assume that positive-result subjects feel well and are not experiencing symptoms, they might conclude that TAA deficiency is not serious or that the test is inaccurate. Because negative-test result subjects are not privy to this information, they may be more likely to conclude that the condition is serious. If minimization occurs primarily when a tested person cannot uncover relevant symptoms, this would suggest that asymptomatic persons should be the least likely to acknowledge the validity of information concerning their heightened susceptibility.

This explanation, of course, presumes that when given the positive test result, subjects in the Jemmott et al. study did not perceive themselves as having symptoms consistent with the diagnosis. A study by Croyle and Sande (1988), however, suggests that this presumption is incorrect. Like the Jemmott et al. study, Croyle and Sande presented subjects with positive and negative test results for TAA deficiency. In addition to measures of perceived seriousness and test accuracy, subjects in this study also completed a symptom checklist after receiving their diagnosis. Subjects were told that symptoms on the list were suspected of being related to TAA deficiency.

The denial effect observed in the Jemmott et al. study was replicated in the Croyle and Sande study: subjects who tested positive for TAA deficiency rated it as less serious and the diagnostic test as less accurate than subjects who tested negative for the condition. In addition, subjects' responses to the symptom checklist indicated that positive test result subjects were able to uncover substantial evidence from memory to confirm the presence of TAA deficiency. Positive-test subjects tended to recall more diagnosis-consistent symptoms than did other subjects. Furthermore, subjects receiving the positive result also recalled more behaviors that were labeled as increasing the risk of TAA deficiency (see Table 7.1).

The Croyle and Sande experiment provided important experimental evidence that risk factor labeling has a direct impact on self-reports of symptoms and health behaviors. These data are also consistent with Leventhal's self-regulation model of illness behavior (Leventhal, Nerenz, & Steele, 1984), which states that individuals assume and seek symmetry between illness labels and symptoms (Leventhal, Meyer, & Nerenz, 1980). The study also provides evidence that is directly inconsistent with one alternative explanation of our findings. Participants do not minimize the seriousness of the risk factor simply because they are unaware of any relevant symptoms.

Table 7.1. Mean Scores on Diagnosis-Consistent Symptom and Risk Behavior Recall Indices as a Function of Test Result

Recall Measure	Test Result	
	Positive	Negative
Symptoms	30.62	20.54
Risk behaviors	101.52	86.79

Source: Croyle & Sande, 1988.
Note: Recall indices were calculated by summing (across 11 diagnosis-consistent symptoms and 9 risk-enhancing behaviors) the number of days during previous month subject reported experiencing the symptom or engaging in the behavior.

Denial and Perceived Treatability

Ditto et al. (1988) took a different approach to examine the motivated nature of reactions to unfavorable test results. Research and theory from the stress and coping literature suggest that denial and other forms of defensiveness are most likely to occur when an individual has no means of immediately reducing the threat (Cohen & Lazarus, 1973; Janis, 1984; Leventhal, 1970). Consequently, two quite different predictions can be made regarding how threat appraisals are likely to be affected by the perception that an unfavorable diagnosis is amenable to treatment. If we adopt the viewpoint of a rational actor, it is reasonable to assume that a treatable disease should be perceived as less threatening than an untreatable one (unless the treatment itself is aversive). From the viewpoint of a person motivated to deny threat, on the other hand, knowledge that the threat can be reduced in the future may allow the individual to more fully acknowledge its immediate seriousness. Following this reasoning, if motivated denial is operating, information that a given disorder is treatable should lead to a paradoxical *increase* in perceived threat among those labeled at risk.

In order to test these competing predictions, Ditto et al. again led some subjects to believe that they had TAA deficiency and some to believe that they did not. Before the risk factor test was conducted, however, half of the subjects were given additional information concerning the treatability of TAA deficiency. Subjects in the treatment-informed condition were told that: "treatment for TAA deficiency is relatively simple and painless. A short-term medication program has been found to correct the deficiency in most people by stimulating TAA production."

The results of the study again provide evidence of motivated denial. Subjects who believed they had the deficiency and were not provided with treatment information made a series of judgments that downplayed the threat represented by their test result. In contrast, positive-result, treatment-informed subjects gave responses that did not differ significantly from the negative-result conditions (see Table 7.2).

In addition to providing additional support for the existence of denial reactions, the Ditto et al. study illustrates the variety of forms such denial reactions can take. As can be seen in Table 7.2, positive-result, treatment-uninformed subjects showed evidence of denial on ratings of the seriousness of both TAA deficiency and pancreatic disease, on estimates of the false-positive rate of the TAA diagnostic test, and on estimates of the probability that TAA deficiency leads to pancreatic disease. Moreover, these subjects' desire not to have the

Table 7.2. Mean Scores on Threat-Related Perceptions as a Function of Test Result and Treatment Information

Dependent Measure	Positive Test Result		Negative Test Result	
	Uninformed	Informed	Uninformed	Informed
TAA test's false-positive rate (%)	24.62	13.95	13.73	12.33
Seriousness of TAA deficiency	22.14	31.43	44.67	39.33
Probability of pancreatic disease given TAA deficiency (%)	21.10	21.67	29.73	43.47
Seriousness of pancreatic disease	55.71	71.90	69.33	60.00
Color of TAA test strip	5.86	6.38	6.73	7.40

Source: Ditto et al., 1988.

Note: The estimated greenness of the TAA strip is on a scale from 1 to 10, where higher numbers indicate darker green. Higher numbers indicate greater perceived seriousness of TAA deficiency and pancreatic disease.

diagnosed condition also manifested itself in perceptual distortion: when shown a color scale and asked to estimate how green their "TAA test strip" had turned, positive-result, treatment-uninformed subjects remembered a less pronounced color reaction than did other subjects.

Denial and Expectations

One last alternative explanation for the motivational account of our denial findings concerns the role of expectations in reactions to medical diagnosis. According to this account, subjects confronted with an unfavorable test result may rate it as less accurate, not because they don't *want* to be sick but rather because they don't *expect* to be sick. Sickness is statistically less common than health, particularly within a college student population. Positive-result subjects may thus discount the accuracy of the test compared with negative-result subjects because the positive result is less expected than the negative result and, consequently, less plausible.

A study by Ditto and Lopez (1992, study 3) addresses this issue. In this study, all subjects were told that they had a relatively rare enzyme condition (present in only 5% of the general population); however, the desirability of this condition was manipulated. Half of the subjects were told, as in previous studies, that the enzyme condition was detrimental to health (increasing one's susceptibility to pancreatic disease). The other half, however, were told that the enzyme condition was actually *beneficial* to health (decreasing one's susceptibility to future pancreatic disease). In addition, half of the subjects completed denial-related dependent measures *after* receiving their diagnostic feedback, whereas the other half answered questions about their diagnosis after hearing the description of the condition but *before* taking the diagnostic test.

The results provided strong support for motivated denial. Subjects asked before receiving their diagnostic feedback rated the test as equally accurate whether the enzyme condition was described as beneficial or detrimental to health. Subjects asked after the diagnostic test, in contrast, rated the test as significantly less accurate when they believed it to indicate a detrimental condition than when they believed it to indicate a beneficial one (see Table 7.3). A similar pattern was shown when subjects were asked to list any recent irregularities in their diet, stress level, etc. that they believed might have affected the accuracy of their test. As can be seen in Table 7.3, like the perceived accuracy ratings, the number of irregularities cited by beneficial-to-health and detrimental-to-health subjects did not differ before receiving their diagnosis. When asked after receiving their diagnosis, however, subjects who believed they had the detrimental condition cited significantly more irregularities that might have affected the accuracy of their test than did subjects diagnosed with the beneficial condition. That these differences are due to the motivational implications of the feedback rather than its consistency with expectations is confirmed by an additional question asked of the pre-diagnosis subjects. When asked before receiving their diagnostic feedback, subjects believing the enzyme condition to be beneficial to health and those believing it to be detrimental to health did not differ in their perceived likelihood of testing positive for the condition.

The Nature of Denial

In addition to providing additional support for the existence of motivational biases in illness appraisals, Ditto and Lopez (1992) offer some

Table 7.3. Mean Perceived Accuracy of Diagnostic Test and Number of Life Irregularities Cited as a Function of Timing of Dependent Measure (Before vs. After Diagnosis) and Desirability of Enzyme Condition (Healthy vs. Unhealthy)

	Before Diagnosis		After Diagnosis	
Dependent Measure	Healthy	Unhealthy	Healthy	Unhealthy
Perceived accuracy of TAA test	6.95	6.68	7.31	5.68
Number of life irregularities cited	1.30	1.21	.55	1.75

Source: Ditto & Lopez (1992).
Note: Higher numbers indicate greater perceived accuracy of TAA test.

specific insights into the nature of these biases. These authors argue that denial and other forms of motivated judgment are a product of the simple fact that more thought is given to information with undesirable implications than to information with desirable implications. That is, a variety of evidence suggests that information that is consistent with a preferred judgment conclusion (e.g., that one is smart, likable, or healthy) receives relatively little cognitive analysis. Because of this uncritical analysis, the validity of information we want to believe is often accepted "at face value." Information that is *inconsistent* with a preferred judgment conclusion on the other hand (e.g., information suggesting that one is not so smart, difficult to like, or ill), seems to trigger relatively extensive, detail-oriented cognitive analysis. Several authors (e.g., Pratto & John, 1991; Schwarz, 1990) have suggested that from an adaptive perspective it makes sense that individuals should be relatively attentive to negative information because it, more often than positive information, requires an immediate behavioral response. However, because the relatively careful analysis given to unwanted information is likely to uncover alternative (and more palatable) explanations for it, a more skeptical view of its validity (i.e., denial) often results.

This view of denial as a kind of "motivated skepticism" has two important implications. First, denial is not an all-or-nothing phenomenon. Individuals confronted with an unfavorable medical diagnosis do not deny its validity and seriousness *in toto*, but rather are simply more likely to view that information as potentially explainable in other, less threatening ways. This is quite consistent with the results of our studies. Positive-result subjects do not view the diagnostic test as completely inaccurate or the diagnosed disorder as completely benign, but only as relatively inaccurate and relatively benign in comparison with negative-result subjects. In fact, the best characterization of our positive-result subjects is that their responses indicate uncertainty about the validity and seriousness of the diagnosis.

The second and related implication is that individuals are quite responsive to negative information—eventually. Most people hold a variety of negative beliefs about themselves (Markus & Wurf, 1987), and even among individuals confronted with diagnoses of cancer, profound denial reactions are clearly the exception rather than the rule (Aitken-Swan & Easson, 1959; Gilbertson & Wangersteen, 1962). Ditto and Lopez suggest that rather than leading individuals to believe whatever they prefer to believe, motivational factors bias judgments more subtly by affecting *the amount of information* required to reach conclusions. People are responsive to incoming information and will generally follow the implications of that information to both preferred and nonpreferred conclusions. However, the greater processing given to undesirable information ought to lead individuals, all else being equal, to reach the point of acceptance somewhat more reluctantly (i.e., after a greater amount or quality of information is received) for nonpreferred conclusions than preferred ones.

To examine the idea that more information is required to reach a nonpreferred conclusion than a preferred one, Ditto and Lopez (1992, study 2) again confronted subjects with either a positive or negative test result for TAA deficiency. In this study, however, this was accomplished by having the TAA test strip remain yellow after contact with saliva rather than turn green. The urinary glucose strips previously used as TAA test strips were replaced with yellow construction paper. When no color reaction was observed after dipping the construction paper in their saliva, half of the subjects perceived this to indicate that they had TAA deficiency (those who would have been negative-result subjects in past studies), and half perceived this to indicate that they did not have TAA deficiency (positive-result subjects in past studies). Subjects were then surreptitiously videotaped while they self-administered the TAA test. All subjects were told that if a color reaction was to take place, it was generally complete within 20 seconds. Subjects were also told that it was important that as soon as they thought their test result was clear, they were to seal their test strip in a provided envelope. The key dependent measure in this study was the amount of time subjects took to decide their test result was complete (i.e., to accept that their test strip was not going to turn green). This was operationalized as the number of seconds between when subjects dipped their test strip in their saliva and when they sealed their test strip in the provided envelope.

All subjects interpreted the test result consistent with instructions. As predicted, however, subjects took almost 30 seconds longer to decide that their test result was complete when they believed that the lack of a color reaction indicated that they had TAA deficiency than when they believed no color reaction to be a negative test result. Stated another way, subjects required more information (i.e., more time) to reach a nonpreferred conclusion (i.e., that they had the risk factor) than to reach a preferred conclusion (i.e., that they did not have the risk factor).

The extra time positive-result subjects required to make their decision was not spent idly. Judges also coded the videotapes for whether subjects "retested" the validity of their diagnosis after observing the initial lack of color reaction. It was found that negative-result subjects typically dipped their test strip once, observed it for a few seconds, and sealed it in the envelope. Positive-result subjects, in contrast, were significantly more likely to engage in retesting behaviors such as repeatedly dipping their test strip in their saliva, testing more than one test strip, testing more than one saliva sample, etc.

One way to view this retesting behavior is as an experimental analogue of the well-known tendency of medical patients to "seek a second opinion." Both the results of this experiment and common sense suggest that individuals are more likely to seek a second opinion when the first opinion is not to their liking. The results may also have implications for home diagnostic testing. Individuals may violate proper testing procedures in order to increase their chance of achieving a favorable result.

Summary

Our studies on college students' reactions to experimentally manipulated diagnoses provide clear support for denial reactions to unfavorable medical test results. Several studies provide converging evidence that the relatively optimistic threat appraisals of positive-result subjects are a function of their desire not to receive this information rather than a rational conclusion based on available symptom or expectancy information. Our studies also suggest that denial is most pronounced when individuals perceive no possibility of a behavioral response to reduce the threat. This suggests that individuals are likely to respond more defensively to a risk factor perceived to be uncontrollable (e.g., one with a genetic basis) than one perceived to be more amenable to change (e.g., one with a behavioral basis). Finally, although the desire to downplay the threat of an unfavorable diagnosis is strong and shows up in many different forms, our data suggest that individuals are ultimately responsive to negative risk factor information. The evidential requirements for accepting an unfavorable diagnosis, however, are stricter than those for accepting a favorable diagnosis and, consequently, clear proof of risk factor status may be necessary before individuals fully acquiesce to its unwanted implications.

THE SOCIAL NATURE OF RISK FACTOR APPRAISAL

Social comparison theory (Festinger, 1954) states that when clear evaluative standards are absent, people evaluate themselves by comparing themselves with others. The effects of prevalence information on risk factor appraisal is a clear example of just this sort of social comparison process. Confronted with an unfamiliar health condition of undetermined seriousness, subjects in the Jemmott et al. (1986) study turned to their immediate social environment for evaluative information. But why should an identically described health disorder be perceived as less serious when it appears to be common than when it appears to be rare?

One answer is that people use perceived prevalence to evaluate the seriousness of health disorders because in many judgmental domains prevalence information is quite predictive of evaluative extremity. Ditto and Jemmott (1989) argue that a basic principle of social comparison is that characteristics are evaluated extremely only to the extent that they differentiate one from others. This is true with both positive and negative characteristics. The ability to run a certain speed or jump a certain distance, for example, is evaluated more positively the fewer the number of other people who are able to match or surpass one's performance. Similarly, a poor performance on some task (e.g., the failure of a math test) is evaluated more negatively the more unusual it is perceived to be. The use of prevalence information to infer evaluation in these domains is quite reasonable. In fact, in these domains the evaluation of performance is almost solely determined by its prevalence.

Ditto and Jemmott argued that based on our experience with domains in which evaluation is socially determined, we come to rely on a *scarcity heuristic* when making all sorts of evaluative judgments. According to this decision-making shortcut, positive stimuli are evaluated more positively and negative stimuli are evaluated more negatively when they are perceived to be rare. When making evaluative judgments in a domain such as health in which evaluation is not socially determined (i.e., the commonness of a health disorder does not determine its seriousness), prevalence information is still used quite automatically to determine evaluative extremity. Ditto and Jemmott (1989) provided evidence for this account in two studies. In both studies, subjects were told about an enzyme condition that either increases or decreases susceptibility to pancreatic disease and is either relatively common or relatively rare. In one study, subjects were told that they had the condition and that either one or four of five fellow subjects had it. In the second study, subjects merely read about the condition. The perceived prevalence of the condition was varied by providing different subjects with different statistical information. Identical results were obtained in both studies: the enzyme condition was evaluated more extremely—more positively when it was said to be beneficial, more negatively when it was said to be detrimental—when it was perceived to be rare.

From these and other data, Ditto and Jemmott argue that the effect of prevalence information on risk factor evaluations is simply one example of our reliance on a quite general evaluation shortcut or heuristic. As is the case with other judgmental heuristics (e.g., Tversky & Kahneman, 1974), the scarcity heuristic is not an altogether unreasonable decision strategy. However, because it relies on a "shortcut" inference process, it may lead to erroneous conclusions in some circumstances (see Ditto & Jemmott, 1989, for a fuller discussion of this point).

Illness Appraisals and Direct Social Influence

Prevalence information is not the only social influence on risk factor appraisals. Appraisals may also be affected more directly by the appraisals stated by others. This is important because prior to seeking formal medical attention, individuals often utilize "lay conferral" networks (e.g., Friedson, 1961) in which the appraisals of family and friends are actively sought in an attempt to interpret uncertain medical situations (Francis, Korsch, & Morris, 1969; Kleinman, Eisenberg, & Good, 1978).

In an initial attempt to capture this more direct form of social influence in the laboratory, Croyle and Hunt (1991) tested subjects for TAA deficiency in the presence of a same-sex confederate who played the role of a second subject. Subjects always tested positive for the deficiency; the test result of the confederate was varied. In addition, for half of the subjects, after receiving the diagnostic information the confederate made a comment that minimized the seriousness of the deficiency ("It doesn't seem like a big deal to me").

Croyle and Hunt found a complex pattern of social influence consistent with the Leventhal et al. (1984) model (see Table 7.4). Leventhal et al. argue that responses to health threats are characterized by two coping processes that occur in parallel. One process involves coping with the threat itself and often is manifested by efforts to reduce risk. A second process involves coping with the fear and other emotional responses to the threatening information. Croyle and Hunt's findings illustrate how these two processes can be affected by different factors. Subjects exposed to the confederate's minimizing comment expressed less *concern* about their diagnosis than did subjects not exposed to the

Table 7.4. Mean Concern and Behavioral Intention Scores as a Function of Confederate's Comment and Test Result

Dependent Measure	No Comment		Minimizing Comment	
	Positive	Negative	Positive	Negative
Concern about TAA deficiency	36.77	45.16	29.23	29.29
Behavioral intention	20.26	23.26	19.69	24.70

Source: From Croyle & Hunt, 1991.

Note: Higher numbers indicate greater concern about TAA deficiency. The health behavior intention score was calculated by summing the ratings of seven behavior intention items. Higher numbers of the behavioral intention index indicate greater intention to engage in behaviors that decrease the risk of developing TAA deficiency.

comment. Subjects' *behavioral intentions* (plans to reduce risk), however, were not affected by the confederate's comments. Rather, intentions to engage in preventive behavior were significantly affected only by the confederate's *diagnosis*. When the confederate also tested positive for the deficiency, subjects reported fewer behavioral intentions than when he or she tested negative. Interestingly, these behavioral intentions were mediated by subjects' perceptions of the prevalence of the deficiency. Mediational analyses revealed that the confederate's positive test result led to perceptions of greater prevalence, which in turn resulted in weaker behavioral intentions. Thus, although this study reveals the importance of more direct forms of social influence on risk factor appraisals, prevalence perceptions again appear to be a key contributing factor.

Illness Appraisals and the False Consensus Bias

Prevalence perceptions not only affect risk factor appraisals but are also affected by them. A commonly observed bias in social psychological research is people's tendency to overestimate the commonness of their behaviors and characteristics. This *false consensus bias* (Ross, Greene, & House, 1977) is also a common finding in our research. Subjects told that they have TAA deficiency estimate its prevalence in the general population to be higher than do subjects told that they do not have TAA deficiency (e.g., Croyle & Sande, 1988; Ditto & Lopez, 1992).

Both motivational and information-processing interpretations of the false consensus bias have been posited (Goethals, 1986; Ross et al., 1977), and which is a better interpretation of the finding in the TAA paradigm is unclear. Given that a common disorder is perceived as less serious than a rare disorder, it is tempting to interpret this bias as another manifestation of defensiveness. Convincing oneself that one's affliction is common should also help convince oneself that it may not be serious. An equally plausible explanation, however, hinges on the differential information available to positive- and negative-result subjects. Positive-result subjects know one person who has the condition (themselves), whereas negative-result subjects do not. Thus, positive-result subjects might reasonably infer from their own ostensible affliction that other people must also be unknowingly afflicted, whereas the basis for this inference is not available to negative-result subjects.

Whatever the genesis of these differential prevalence perceptions, once established they are likely to have some important implications. For example, unlike some of the other biases we have documented in college students' judgments, the false consensus bias is also manifested by physicians. Jemmott, Croyle, and Ditto (1988) sent questionnaires to 65 practicing physicians asking them about their experience with and beliefs about 13 well-known health disorders (e.g., migraine headaches, viral pneumonia). Physicians' estimates of the prevalence of the health disorders in the general population revealed a false consensus bias. Physicians who had experienced a given health problem gave higher estimates of its prevalence than did physicians who had never experienced the problem. For example, physicians who had had herpes simplex virus infection of the lips estimated its population prevalence at 52%. Physicians who had never experienced the same problem estimated its prevalence to be only 15%.

These findings have implications for diagnostic reasoning. Medical textbooks suggest that physicians consider the prevalence of a particular disorder both in general and within a specific subpopulation when developing diagnostic hypotheses (Cutler, 1979; Petersdorf et al., 1983). Several studies have also shown that diagnostic reasoning is biased toward hypothesis confirmation (Elstein, Shulman, & Sprafka, 1978; Snyder, 1984). Putting these two facts together, it seems possible that physicians who believe that a particular disorder is prevalent because they have had it themselves may be more likely to entertain that disorder as a diagnostic hypothesis and, consequently, more likely to decide on it as the ultimate diagnosis. In the case of risk factor labeling, this suggests that physicians' beliefs concerning their own risk factor status may have a direct or indirect influence on their identification of important risk factors in their patients. The extent to which physicians' personal experience with health disorders influences their diagnostic strategies and ultimate diagnoses is an important topic for future research.

Summary

Our research suggests that risk factor appraisal has important social psychological aspects. Appraisals of the seriousness of a risk factor are affected by the appraisals offered by others. That this effect was demonstrated in a laboratory context with the appraisal of a stranger suggests that this effect is likely to be considerably more pronounced when such appraisals are offered by a good friend or family member. Seriousness judgments are also affected by the perceived prevalence of the risk factor. Although this may not at first glance seem unreasonable, the heuristic nature of this judgment strategy creates the possibility of misperceptions. One simple example of this in our studies is the fact that subjects readily base their prevalence estimates (and consequently their seriousness appraisals) on data gathered from very small samples. Even if the prevalence of a condition was perfectly predictive of its severity, a prevalence estimate based on a sample of one (Croyle & Hunt, 1991) or even five (Ditto & Jemmott, 1989; Jemmott et al., 1986) may be highly unrepresentative of the actual prevalence rate in the general population. Finally, our studies reveal a false census bias in risk factor appraisals. Although the specific causes of this bias are unclear, it is revealed by both physicians and laypersons and may have important consequences for both populations' subsequent decision making.

THE GENERALIZABILITY ISSUE

The preceding sections have reviewed some of the insights gained about risk factor appraisals from a series of laboratory experiments. The strengths of laboratory experimentation are clear. The ability of our experimental procedure to isolate the causal contribution of specific factors to specific aspects of risk factor appraisals cannot be matched with more naturalistic methodologies. And yet, the weaknesses of laboratory experimentation are equally clear. The purchase price of internal validity is the greater assumptions that must be made about external validity. In the case of our TAA experiments, the question concerns the degree to which the phenomena we observe in our laboratory simulation generalize to people's appraisals of actual risk factors in actual risk factor screening situations.

In the sections that follow we discuss several of the most commonly mentioned generalization issues that arise concerning the results of our TAA studies. Where possible, we then describe data to address each issue. To foreshadow our conclusions, considerable data supports the generalizability of the basic findings obtained with the TAA enzyme paradigm.

Psychological Reactions to Well-Known Risk Factors

Perhaps the most often expressed concern about the TAA enzyme paradigm is its use of a fictitious and therefore completely unfamiliar risk factor. The assumption is that individuals might respond quite differently when confronted with evidence of some more familiar health condition.

Two different lines of research, however, suggest that the basic phenomena that are observed in reaction to TAA deficiency can be observed in reactions to actual risk factors as well. The first examines judgments about actual health conditions within a survey format. The second is a series of studies in which individuals are given experimentally engineered feedback about their status on some actual risk factor.

Jemmott et al. (1988, study 1) asked college students to make a series of judgments about 12 well-known health disorders. Three major findings emerged. First, consistent with the minimization effect found in laboratory TAA studies, individuals who had experienced a given disorder rated that disorder as significantly less serious than did individuals who had not experienced that disorder. Second, consistent with the finding that prevalence information affects seriousness judgments, the average correlation between students' estimates of the prevalence of a given disorder in the general population and their rating of its seriousness was significant and negative. That is, the more common a given disorder was perceived to be, the less serious it was perceived to be and vice versa (see also Jemmott et al., 1986). Finally, a false consensus effect was also observed. Individuals who had experienced a given disorder gave higher estimates of its prevalence in the general population than did individuals with no experience with the disorder. Although the causal interpretation of the observed relationships is less clear in this correlational data than in the experimental data, the converging findings from the two approaches provide strong evidence for generalizability.

The results from experimental studies tell a similar tale. Croyle, Sun, and Louie (1993) gave subjects a standard blood cholesterol screening test and randomly assigned them to receive a total cholesterol reading that was either in the clearly low-risk range (174 mg/dl) or one that was borderline high (224 mg/dl). (Subjects were given their actual cholesterol readings during debriefing.) Appraisals of the cholesterol feedback were remarkably similar to appraisals of randomized TAA feedback. Subjects receiving the borderline-high feedback rated high cholesterol as a less serious threat to health, gave higher estimates of its population prevalence, and viewed the cholesterol test as less accurate than did subjects receiving the more desirable reading.

McCaul, Thiesse-Duffy, and Wilson (1991) found very similar results in appraisals of bogus gum disease feedback. Subjects volunteered to have a standard gum health exam at a campus dental office. After completing the examination, subjects were randomly assigned to receive one of three diagnoses from the dental hygienist. One third were told that they had gum disease, one third that they were at risk for gum disease, and the final third that they did not have gum disease. Subjects' postdiagnosis appraisals were consistent with previous research. Subjects told they had gum disease rated it as a more common condition than did subjects receiving at-risk feedback, who in turn perceived it as more common than did subjects receiving no-disease feedback. Disease and at-risk subjects also rated gum disease as a less serious threat to health than did no-disease subjects. Finally, the "paradoxical" relationship between denial and confirmatory symptom reporting (Croyle & Sande, 1988) was also replicated. Subjects returned to the dental office to answer additional questions 2 days after receiving the diagnostic feedback. Subjects assigned the disease and at-risk feedback reported experiencing more bleeding from the gums (which they were told was a symptom of gum disease) than did no-disease subjects.*

Appraisals of experimentally manipulated blood pressure feedback also confirm findings from the TAA enzyme paradigm. In two experiments, Croyle (1990) measured subjects' blood pressure and then randomly assigned them to receive either high blood pressure feedback (140/97) or normal blood pressure feedback (110/80). The results of the studies mirror those of studies using the TAA paradigm: subjects receiving the high blood pressure feedback rated high blood pressure as a less serious threat to health than did subjects receiving normal blood pressure feedback.

Confirmatory symptom reporting has also been demonstrated within the context of blood pressure testing. Baumann, Cameron,

---

*Interestingly, the three groups of subjects did not differ in their perceptions of the accuracy of the diagnostic test. McCaul et al. argue that this is likely due to the fact that the professionally administered gum exam was perceived to be a highly valid indicator of gum disease. Consequently, it may have been difficult for disease and at-risk subjects to plausibly entertain the notion that the test result might be inaccurate.

Zimmerman, and Leventhal (1989) randomly assigned subjects normal and high blood pressure feedback and found that high blood pressure subjects were more likely than normal blood pressure subjects to report symptoms laypersons commonly associate with hypertension. This effect was especially pronounced when high blood pressure subjects attributed their elevated reading to stress.

This latter finding illustrates that important insights can be gained from research on actual risk factors like hypertension that are unlikely to emerge from TAA research alone. A person's mental representations of the causes, consequences, and time course of health disorders have been shown to play an important role in appraisal processes (Ditto et al., 1988; Skelton & Croyle, 1991). Much of this research has concerned mental representations of hypertension (e.g., Meyer, Leventhal, & Guttman, 1985). Building on this nonexperimental work, research on experimentally manipulated blood pressure feedback has confirmed that mental representations can both affect appraisals and be affected by them.

Meyer et al. (1985), for example, have shown that mental representations of hypertension are characterized by one of three types of beliefs concerning the time course of the disorder. Some people view it as an acute condition, others as a cyclical condition that comes and goes, and still others adhere to the medically accepted chronic view of the disorder. Croyle (1990) found that which one of these views an individual ascribes to can be affected by diagnostic feedback. After they received their blood pressure results, subjects in Croyle's second experiment were asked whether they believed hypertension was an acute, cyclical, or chronic condition. Subjects told their blood pressure was high were less likely than low blood pressure subjects to endorse a chronic model of hypertension (see also Baumann et al., 1989). The findings also showed that minimization among subjects receiving the high blood pressure feedback was related to mental representations. Minimization occurred only among subjects who believed that hypertension was an acute or cyclical problem.

A study by Croyle and Williams (1991) makes a similar point regarding the interplay between mental representations and illness appraisals. The study examined the role of what Croyle and Williams call "illness stereotypes" in reactions to medical diagnoses. First, a small survey was conducted; it found that individuals who rated high blood pressure as a less serious threat to health also tended to associate the disorder with positive personal characteristics (e.g., professional employment, high intelligence). This relationship was then confirmed in a laboratory experiment. Subjects read information about high blood pressure that stated that it was associated either with undesirable personality characteristics, such as the tendency to panic under pressure, or with desirable personality characteristics leading to academic and professional success. When subjects were subsequently given false feedback indicating that their blood pressure was high, those given the positive stereotype information rated high blood pressure as a less serious threat to health and reported more hypertension-related symptoms than did subjects given the negative stereotype information.

In summary, both correlational and experimental research on appraisals of actual risk factors confirm the results found in the TAA enzyme paradigm. Minimization of risk factor seriousness and diagnostic test accuracy, the relationship between perceived prevalence and perceived seriousness, the false consensus bias, and confirmatory symptom reporting have all been demonstrated with appraisals of actual risk factors.

Research examining the impact of randomized feedback concerning actual risk factors, however, has not been limited to replications of phenomena discovered in the laboratory. Experimental studies using actual risk factors can also lead to novel insights regarding the determinants of risk factor appraisals. Although many of the important psychological processes underlying threat appraisal operate similarly across disease domains, each risk factor or disease also has unique features that raise some unique psychological issues. This is illustrated by the study of hypertension screening described earlier (Croyle, 1990). Another example is provided by the many tests now under development in the field of human genetics. Clearly, feedback on genetic tests have family and family-planning implications that nongenetic tests do not have (see Croyle & Lerman, Chapter 2). As field studies of new screening technologies begin to yield findings regarding psychosocial effects, the need to isolate and clarify these effects will influence the course of basic laboratory research on appraisal.

Diagnostic Context

Another obvious concern about the generalizability of results from the TAA enzyme paradigm is the artificial context within which subjects receive their diagnostic feedback. Is self-administering a saliva test in a psychological research lab the same as receiving diagnostic feedback from a medical professional?

We have two answers to that question. The first is that several studies have shown that similar patterns of risk factor appraisals are observed when the diagnostic test is professionally administered as when the test is self-administered. All of the studies cited above examining reactions to blood pressure and cholesterol feedback were administered by someone other than the subject. In addition, two studies have been done in which the test was conducted at a university healthy facility. Croyle and Sande (1988) tested students for TAA deficiency at a student infirmary. An experimenter in a nurse's uniform conducted the test. McCaul et al. (1991) tested subjects at the campus dental office. Testing was done by a professional dental hygienist. All of these studies produced results virtually identical to those found when subjects self-administer the TAA saliva test.

The second answer to the question is that reactions to self-administered and professionally administered tests might indeed show important differences. This does not, however, make reactions to self-diagnosis uninteresting. Quite the contrary, the recent proliferation of over-the-counter diagnostic tests makes reactions to self-administered tests an increasingly important topic of study. At-home assays can now be conducted for a variety of conditions from pregnancy and ovulation to the examination of plasma or urinary glucose levels. More such tests are likely to be available in the near future. The TAA paradigm would seem a particularly good analogue of these types of self-administered diagnostic tests.

One potential difference between reactions to professionally administered and self-administered diagnostic tests concerns the level of ambiguity surrounding the meaning of the test result. Without a medical professional present, the individual self-administering a diagnostic test may be left with considerable uncertainty regarding interpretation of the test result. The more uncertainty, the more room for biased processing of the diagnostic information to operate. Croyle and Sande (1988), for example, found that when subjects were led to be relatively uncertain regarding the meaning of an unfavorable test result (i.e., that it was 75% accurate), they were *less* rather than more likely to request a second, more definite diagnostic test than subjects who were led to be more certain of the test's diagnostic value (i.e., that it was 95% accurate).

Another negative consequence of uncertainty is that it may be unsettling even when the test result is seemingly favorable. Cioffi (1991), in fact, has suggested that individuals may find a diagnosis of "uncertain wellness" uniquely troubling. Utilizing the TAA enzyme paradigm, Cioffi used instructions to manipulate both the favorability of the test result (deficiency or no deficiency) as well as its clarity (the color reaction in the test strip either clearly matched the color expected for the diagnosis or was a color that was at the perceptual midpoint between the diagnosis and an "invalid" reading). Her results indicated that, compared with subjects receiving the other diagnoses, subjects receiving the unclear-well diagnosis reported more concern about their health, heightened perceived vulnerability to pancreatic disease, and a strong desire for treatment. Cioffi suggests that the unclear-well diagnosis may be emotionally unsettling because, while indicating some possibility of illness, it does not initiate the type of self-protective mechanisms typically observed in reaction to more unambiguous negative diagnoses. Consequently, the subjects are left with fear and uncertainty regarding their health status without the emotional buffer provided by threat-minimizing beliefs such as perceiving the looming disease as benign and/or the diagnostic test as potentially invalid.

In summary, experimental studies have shown that people respond similarly to risk factor information whether it is professionally administered or self-administered and whether or not the test is conducted in a formal medical context. Future studies might more specifically pursue differences in reactions to professionally administered and self-administered tests as well as examining the unique properties of the increasingly more common phenomenon of self-diagnosis.

Immediate versus Delayed Reactions

Ethical concerns generally restrict the use of the TAA enzyme paradigm to the examination of immediate reactions to risk factor information. Immediate reactions to unfavorable risk factor information are theoretically interesting because the conflicting emotional and problem-focused coping demands placed on the individual are most intense at this time. Many important decisions, however, may not be made until some time after the risk factor information is initially received and "digested." Risk factor appraisals may change over time (Lazarus & Folkman, 1984; Lehman, Wortman, & Williams, 1987; Suls & Fletcher, 1985) as the individual gathers and integrates new information about the condition.

One study, however, suggests that the minimization response observed immediately after the receipt of diagnostic information may persist for at least a matter of days. McCaul et al. (1991) measured subjects' appraisals of gum disease immediately after receiving diagnostic feedback and again 2 days later. Appraisals measured after 2 days were virtually identical to those measured immediately. Subjects who were told they had gum disease still rated it as significantly less serious and more prevalent than did subjects in the at-risk and no-disease conditions 2 days after initially receiving the diagnosis. Two days is a relatively brief period of time, particularly in comparison to the time frames experienced in real-life coping situations. However, these data do show that the minimization effect observed immediately after receiving diagnostic information is not merely a transitory effect induced within a brief psychology experiment.

Reactions to Serious Medical Conditions

Ethical concerns also preclude experimental studies from examining reactions to extremely serious medical conditions. Although the TAA enzyme paradigm is likely to be a relatively close analogue to cholesterol and hypertension screening, its generalizability to appraisals of more immediately life-threatening medical conditions is more tenuous.

At one level, the TAA paradigm seems most likely to *underestimate* the effects observed in response to serious medical conditions. This would seem especially likely in terms of defensive reactions like minimization. Indeed, one fascinating aspect of the TAA enzyme paradigm is that defensive appraisals like those more typically expected in response to life-threatening conditions such as cancer or myocardial infarction can be reliably observed in subjects' reactions to a relatively benign and unfamiliar risk factor.

Other determinants of risk factor appraisals, however, may be less likely to operate when an individual is confronted with a clearly serious medical condition. The operation of judgmental biases and heuristics is most apparent under conditions of uncertainty (Kahneman, Slovic, & Tversky, 1982). To the extent that clear information is available about any judgmental dimension, therefore, judgments along this dimension are less likely to be affected by such extraneous factors. As just one example, the perceived prevalence of a condition is unlikely to affect seriousness judgments to the extent that other, more compelling evidence of the condition's seriousness is also available (Ditto & Jemmott, 1989).

Individual Differences in Reactions to Risk Factor Information

So far, our discussion of generalizability has focused on the degree to which similar reactions are observed across variations in aspects of the diagnostic situation (e.g., type and seriousness of the diagnosed risk factor, the context of diagnosis). A second dimension on which generalizability can be discussed, however, concerns the degree to which similar reactions are observed across individuals with different personalities. That is, to what extent do individual differences exist in how people appraise risk factor information?

One issue that can be subsumed under the general rubric of individual differences concerns the extent to which conclusions based on the responses of college students can be taken as representative of the broader population. In all of our experimental studies of risk factor screening employing the TAA enzyme paradigm, the subjects have been college students. Both ethical and logistical concerns make college students the most attractive population for study. Generalizing from the responses of young, predominantly healthy college students to the broader population, however, must be done with great caution. Empirical support for any such generalizations must be provided before they can be made with confidence.

Several lines of reasoning, however, suggest that the differences between college students' responses to risk factor information and those of other segments of the population might be less pronounced than one might initially imagine. First, many of the hypotheses tested by our experimental studies were originally derived from observations of older patients' reactions to real health disorders (e.g., Lipowski, 1970; Visotsky et al., 1961; Zola, 1966). Thus, there are already data to suggest that these phenomena are observed in the broader population. Second, although a few studies of health-related judgments have shown age to be an important factor (e.g., Leventhal & Prohaska, 1986; Prohaska, Keller, Leventhal, & Leventhal, 1987), other studies have found that risk minimization is pervasive in both college student and community samples (e.g., Croyle, Sun, & Louie, 1993; Weinstein, 1982; 1987). Third, to the extent that risk factor information is received unaccompanied by experienced symptomatology, college students' relative lack of symptomatology does not pose a serious problem in terms of generalization.

Finally, more indirect evidence for the generalizability of results obtained from college students comes from the fact that several initial studies have shown little relationship between individual difference variables and risk factor appraisals. Croyle et al. (1993) found subjects' appraisals of cholesterol feedback to be unrelated to either previously measured self-esteem (indexed by the Rosenberg [1965] self-esteem scale) or monitoring vs. blunting coping style (indexed by the Miller [1987; Miller, Brody, & Summerton, 1988] Behavioral Style Scale). Ditto et al. (1988) reported no significant correlations between scores on the facilitation-inhibition scale (a shortened version of the repression-sensitization scale developed by Ullman, 1962) and minimization reactions. Moore and Ditto (1991) found minimization of positive test results to be unaffected by subjects' scores on the Whiteley Index (a measure of hypochondriacal beliefs developed by Pilowsky, 1967). And Croyle, Barger, and Sun (1992) reported that repressive coping style was unrelated to seriousness appraisals of TAA enzyme deficiency. Less formally, several other individual difference scales have been included in TAA studies conducted in our laboratories, such as the Life Orientation Test (Scheier & Carver, 1985) and the Marlowe-Crowne Social Desirability Scale (Crowne & Marlowe, 1964), and no significant relationships with risk factor appraisals have been observed. Gender has shown no consistent relationship with any aspect of risk factor appraisals.

In summary then, results from several initial studies suggest that risk factor appraisals are relatively unaffected by several measures of conceptually relevant individual differences. Research on this issue, however, has just begun. Although the increased application of risk factor screening to college students makes them an important population in their own right, further research is needed to determine any differences in reactions between this and other demographic groups. The individual difference variables examined to date have been those whose theoretical relationship to reactions to threatening information have been most clear. Many other personality and attitude dimensions, however, have yet to be examined. Finally, our initial studies have been primarily concerned with individual differences in immediate cognitive appraisals. The receipt of unfavorable diagnostic information is likely to be such a salient situation that the effects of any individual difference variables may be temporarily overwhelmed (e.g., Kenrick, McCreath, Govern, King, & Bordin, 1990). Individual differences may emerge more clearly in longer-term cognitive and behavioral reactions to risk factor information.

Generalizing from Appraisal to Behavior

Experimental work on psychological reactions to risk factor information has been predominantly concerned with cognitive appraisals. Much less attention has been paid to obtaining measures of subjects' behavioral responses. For the most part, this emphasis on appraisal processes reflects our belief that the cognitive underpinnings of illness behavior are a crucial and understudied topic. Still, the individual's behavioral response to risk factor information—whether the individual seeks treatment or information, whether he or she enacts prescribed changes in behavior—remains of paramount practical importance. And while cognitive appraisals may provide important insights into an individual's likely behavioral response, research in social and personality psychology has clearly demonstrated that the cognition-behavior relationship is anything but simple (Quattrone, 1985; Schuman & Johnson, 1976; Wicker, 1969). Thus, a final issue that must be discussed is the nature of the relationship between cognitive appraisals of risk factor information and subsequent behavior.

Behavioral measures are not the strong suit of experimental research in social and personality psychology. However, our experiments have typically included "behavioroid" measures of some type. Behavioroid measures are those that assess behavioral intention or choice. The simplest (and consequently, least compelling) measure has been simply asking subjects to indicate on a scale their interest in obtaining additional information about TAA deficiency and pancreatic disease (Ditto et al., 1988). Several other studies have asked subjects to indicate their *intentions* (Ajzen & Fishbein, 1980) of engaging in a variety of preventive or reactive behaviors (Croyle & Hunt, 1991; Croyle, et al., 1993). Finally, several studies have used a method in which subjects are offered the opportunity to review any or all of a series of informational services about TAA deficiency (a free pamphlet, a booklet costing 50¢, a free physical examination) (Ditto & Jemmott, 1989; Jemmott et al., 1986). Subjects indicate which (if any) of these services they wish to receive and the number of services requested is used as the dependent measure.

Studies utilizing these types of behavioral measures have shown that in some instances the appraisal-behavior relationship is relatively straightforward. Ditto and Jemmott (1989) found that the effect of prevalence information on perceptions of seriousness translated quite directly into behavior. Subjects led to believe that they had a rare enzyme condition not only perceived it to be more serious than subjects led to believe the condition was common but were also significantly more likely to sign up to receive additional information about their condition. Behavioral intention data from Croyle and Hunt (1991) also confirm that conditions perceived to be rare provoke a relatively vigorous behavioral response.

Studies examining denial reactions to unfavorable diagnostic information, however, suggest a more complex appraisal-behavior relationship. The simple assumption when considering denial reactions is that the lowered appraisals of threat offered by positive-result subjects should manifest themselves in similarly lower levels of behavioral responding. Denial, in other words, is often viewed as a maladaptive response (e.g., Haan, 1977) and one that is likely to interfere with adaptive behavioral responses to threatening risk factor information.

The results of several of our experimental studies, however, have shown this not to be the case. Jemmott et al. (1986) for example, found that although positive-result subjects rated TAA deficiency as less serious and the TAA diagnostic test as less accurate than did negative-result subjects, they also requested significantly more additional information about TAA deficiency than did negative-result subjects. Croyle et al. (1993) show a similar pattern in reactions to cholesterol feedback using a measure of behavioral intentions. Finally, the pattern of data found by Ditto et al. (1988) is particularly telling. These investigators found a more pronounced denial reaction when positive-result subjects believed TAA deficiency to be untreatable than when they perceived it to be treatable. Still, positive-result, untreatable subjects showed interest in additional information about TAA deficiency and pancreatic disease that was just as high as positive-result, treatable subjects and significantly higher than that expressed by negative-result subjects. In other words, the more pronounced denial reactions observed by subjects perceiving their affliction as untreatable showed no evidence of dampening interest in additional information. This is particularly impressive in light of the fact that additional information is probably perceived as less likely to be useful if one's condition is not thought to be amenable to treatment.

This seemingly paradoxical relationship between denial and ameliorative behavior is reminiscent of the relationship between denial and symptom reporting (Croyle & Sande, 1988; McCaul et al., 1991). Both findings are consistent with Lazarus and Folkman's (1984) distinction between emotion-focused and problem-focused coping and Leventhal et al.'s (1984) self-regulation theory of illness behavior. Both of these models conceive of the coping process stimulated by a health threat as simultaneously proceeding along two parallel pathways. Lazarus and Folkman (1984) make a distinction between attempts to cope with the emotional upset resulting from the perception of threat (emotion-focused coping) and attempts to cope with the threatening agent itself (problem-focused coping). These two processes are thought to operate independently. Leventhal's self-regulation model similarly postulates a two-pathway coping process. One pathway corresponds to emotion-focused coping and involves "the creation of an emotional response to the problem and the development of a coping plan for the management of emotion." The second pathway corresponds to problem-focused coping and involves "the creation of an objective view or representation of an illness threat and the development of a coping plan to manage that threat" (p. 220). In Leventhal et al.'s view, as in Lazarus and Folkman's, these processes are thought to operate semi-independently.

The denial processes observed in our studies are best conceived of as attempts to attenuate emotional upset. The search for relevant symptomatology and the construction of an adaptive behavioral response, on the other hand, represent the problem-focused pathway. Consistent with both theoretical models, our data suggest that these two processes operate independently. At the same time that the individual is minimizing the threat represented by the risk factor information in an attempt to control emotional upset, she or he is attempting to construct an accurate representation of the illness threat (symptom search) and taking active behavioral measures to cope with it. Additional evidence of independence comes from the fact that the two coping pathways appear to be affected by different variables (Croyle & Hunt, 1991).

An important implication of this separate pathways view of illness behavior is that the defensive processes that are initiated by unfavorable test results may not deserve the negative connotations that are often placed on them. Rather than disrupting adaptive problem-focused coping attempts, casting a threatening situation in a relatively benign light may actually facilitate such attempts by keeping potentially disruptive emotional responses in check (Cohen & Lazarus, 1979; Lazarus, 1983; Taylor, 1983). This view of denial is consistent not only with data from the TAA paradigm, but also with other data suggesting an association between coping attempts characterized by denial and positive postsurgical outcomes (e.g., Cohen & Lazarus, 1973).

This more charitable view of denial is also consistent with Ditto and Lopez's (1992) characterization of motivational biases in judgment. According to this view, denial is rarely a total rejection of threatening information, but rather a kind of "motivated skepticism" fueled by a heightened sensitivity to alternative explanations for unwanted information. Thus, the individual confronted with an unfavorable test result does not walk away convinced of its invalidity, but rather with a sense that the test result is potentially "confounded," and with some hope intact that a more agreeable interpretation is possible. This view of denial also removes the paradoxical nature from the appraisal-behavior relationship. Seeking treatment or information about a condition is paradoxical only if the individual is convinced that he or she is healthy.

In summary, more research is needed on the relationship between cognitive appraisals of risk factor information and subsequent behavioral responses. Our data suggest that this relationship is not necessarily a simple one. This is in large part due to the multiple coping demands faced by individuals confronted with an unfavorable diagnosis. Emotional and practical concerns must be dealt with simultaneously, resulting in a complex pattern of affective, cognitive, and behavioral responses. One implication from our data that is consistent with prominent theoretical models of illness behavior is that defensive biases in appraisal are not necessarily maladaptive. Denial processes may serve the important function of controlling potentially disruptive emotions. If this is the case, then disrupting this natural coping mechanism may have undesirable consequences.

CONCLUSIONS

This chapter reviewed experimental evidence on reactions to risk factor information. The majority of the studies reported utilized a research paradigm that was developed to investigate the psychological processes underlying the appraisal of risk factor test results by randomizing subjects to different test result conditions. Almost all of the studies have used college students as subjects and have focused on short-term reactions to risk information.

As a whole, the research provides strong and consistent evidence that initial appraisals are characterized by threat minimization. Subjects who receive test results indicative of a risk factor appraise it as less serious and the risk factor test as less accurate than do those who receive favorable test results. Subjects who are told they have a risk factor later perceive it as relatively common, but they also seek relevant information and express behavioral intentions that suggest the development of a plan for actively coping with the threat.

The research also provides consistent evidence that risk factor appraisals are affected by social factors. Both perceptions of the commonness of the risk factor and appraisals of the risk factor offered by others affect perceptions of its seriousness. Seriousness appraisals subsequently determine individuals' behavioral response to the risk factor information.

Substantial convergent evidence shows that findings regarding appraisal phenomena observed in the laboratory can be generalized to non-laboratory settings. The findings from studies examining college students' reactions to fictitious risk factors have been replicated in studies utilizing real screening tests (e.g., cholesterol and blood pressure) and more diverse adult populations.

Laboratory experiments on risk factor testing cannot provide answers to all of the important questions concerning labeling effects. We do believe, however, that controlled studies of randomized feedback provide a critical and unique contribution to the body of work on the psychosocial impact of risk factor testing.

NOTE

Preparation of this manuscript was supported by grants from the National Institute of Mental Health grant (MH43097) and the Agency for Health Care Policy Research (HS 06660) awarded to the second author.

REFERENCES

Aitken-Swan, J., & Easson, E. C. (1959). Reactions of cancer patients on being told their diagnosis. *British Medical Journal, 1*, 779–783.

Ajzen, I., & Fishbein, M. (1980). *Understanding attitudes and predicting social behavior.* Englewood Cliffs, NJ: Prentice-Hall.

Aronson, E., Ellsworth, P. C., Carlsmith, J. M., & Gonzales, M. H. (1990). Methods of research in social psychology (2nd ed.). New York: McGraw-Hill.

Baumann, L. J., Cameron, L. D., Zimmerman, R. S., & Leventhal, H. (1989). Illness representations and matching labels with symptoms. *Health Psychology, 8*, 449–469.

Cioffi, D. (1991). Asymmetry of doubt in medical self-diagnosis: The ambiguity of "uncertain wellness." *Journal of Personality and Social Psychology, 61*, 969–980.

Cohen, F., & Lazarus, R. S. (1973). Active coping processes, coping dispositions, and recovery from surgery. *Psychosomatic Medicine, 35*, 357–389.

———. (1979). Coping with the stresses of illness. In G. Stone, F. Cohen, & N. Adler (Eds.), *Health psychology: A handbook* (pp. 217–254). San Francisco: Jossey-Bass.

Crowne, D. P., & Marlowe, D. (1964). *The approval motive: Studies in evaluative dependence.* New York: Wiley.

Croyle, R. T. (1990). Biased appraisal of high blood pressure. *Preventive Medicine, 19*, 40–44.

Croyle, R. T., Barger, S. D., & Sun, Y. (1992). Repressive coping style and appraisal of health threat. Unpublished data, University of Utah.

Croyle, R. T., & Ditto, P. H. (1990). Illness cognition and behavior: An experimental approach. *Journal of Behavioral Medicine, 13*, 31–52.

Croyle, R. T., & Hunt, J. R. (1991). Coping with health threat: Social influence processes in reactions to medical test results. *Journal of Personality and Social Psychology, 60*, 382–389.

Croyle, R. T., & Sande, G. N. (1988). Denial and confirmatory search: Paradoxical consequences of medical diagnoses. *Journal of Applied Social Psychology, 18*, 473–490.

Croyle, R. T., Sun, Y., & Louie, D. H. (1993). Psychological minimization of choles-terol test results: Moderators of appraisal in college students and commu-nity residents. *Health Psychology, 12,* 503–507.

Croyle, R. T., & Williams, K. D. (1991). Reactions to medical diagnosis: The role of illness stereotypes. *Basic and Applied Social Psychology, 12,* 227–241.

Cutler, P. (1979). *Problem solving in clinical medicine: From data to diagnosis.* Balti-more: Williams & Wilkins.

Ditto, P. H., & Jemmott, J. B., III (1989). From rarity to evaluative extremity: Effects of prevalence information on evaluations of positive and negative characteristics. *Journal of Personality and Social Psychology, 57,* 16–26.

Ditto, P. H., Jemmott, J. B., III, & Darley, J. M. (1988). Appraising the threat of illness: A mental representational approach. *Health Psychology, 7,* 183–200.

Ditto, P. H., & Lopez, D. F. (1992). Motivated skepticism: The use of differential decision criteria for preferred and nonpreferred conclusions. *Journal of Personality and Social Psychology, 63,* 568–584.

Elstein, A. S., Shulman, L. S., & Sprafka, S. A. (1978). *Medical problem solving: An analysis of clinical reasoning.* Cambridge, MA: Harvard University Press.

Erdeyli, M. H. (1974). A new look at the new look: Perceptual defense and vigi-lance. *Psychological Review, 81,* 1–25.

Festinger, L. (1954). A theory of social comparison processes. *Human Relations, 7,* 117–140.

Francis, V., Korsch, B. M., & Morris, M. J. (1969). Gaps in doctor-patient communi-cations: Patients' response to medical advice. *New England Journal of Medi-cine, 280,* 535–540.

Friedson, E. (1961). *Patients' view of medical practice.* New York: Russell Sage Foundation.

Gilbertson, V. A., & Wangersteen, O. H. (1962). Should the doctor tell the patient that the disease is cancer? In *The physician and the total care of the cancer patient* (pp. 80–85). New York: American Cancer Society.

Goethals, G. R. (1986). Fabricating and ignoring social reality: Self-serving esti-mates of consensus. In J. Olson, C. P. Herman, & M. P. Zanna (Eds.), *Relative deprivation and social comparison: The Ontario symposium* (Vol. 4, pp. 135–158). Hillsdale, NJ: Erlbaum.

Haan, N. (1977). *Coping and defending.* New York: Academic Press.

Hackett, T. P., & Cassem, N. H. (1969). Factors contributing to delay in responding to the signs and symptoms of acute myocardial infarction. *American Journal of Cardiology, 24,* 651–658.

Janis, I. L. (1958). *Psychological stress.* New York: Wiley.

———. (1984). Improving adherence to medical recommendations: Prescriptive hypotheses derived from recent research in social psychology. In A. Baum, S. Taylor, & J. Singer (Eds.), *Handbook of psychology and health* (Vol. 4): *Social psychological aspects of health* (pp. 113–148). Hillsdale, NJ: Erlbaum.

Jemmott, J. B., III, Ditto, P. H., & Croyle, R. T. (1986). Judging health status: Effects of perceived prevalence and personal relevance. *Journal of Personality and Social Psychology, 50,* 899–905.

———. (1988). Commonsense epidemiology: Self-based judgments from layper-sons and physicians. *Health Psychology, 7,* 55–73.

Kahneman, D., Slovic, P., & Tversky, A. (1982). *Judgment under uncertainty: Heuris-tics and biases.* New York: Cambridge University Press.

Kenrick, D. T., McCreath, H. E., Govern, J., King, R., & Bordin, J. (1990). Person-environment intersections: Everyday settings and common trait dimensions. *Journal of Personality and Social Psychology, 58,* 685–698.

Kleinman, A., Eisenberg, L., & Good, B. (1978). Culture, illness, and care. *Annals of Internal Medicine, 88,* 251–258.

Kubler-Ross, E. (1969). *On death and dying.* New York: Macmillan.

Lazarus, R. S. (1983). The costs and benefits of denial. In S. Breznitz (Ed.), *The denial of stress* (pp. 1–30). New York: International Universities Press.

Lazarus, R. S., & Folkman, S. (1984). *Stress, appraisal, and coping.* New York: Springer-Verlag.

Lehman, D. R., Wortman, C. B., & Williams, A. F. (1987). Long-term effects of losing a spouse or child in a motor vehicle crash. *Journal of Personality and Social Psychology, 52,* 218–231.

Leventhal, E. A., & Prohaska, T. R. (1986). Age, symptom interpretation, and health behavior. *Journal of the American Geriatric Society, 34,* 185–191.

Leventhal, H. (1970). Findings and theory in the study of fear communications. In L. Berkowitz (Ed.), *Advances in experimental social psychology* (Vol. 5, pp. 119–186). New York. Academic Press.

Leventhal, H., Meyer, D., & Nerenz, D. (1980). The commonsense representation of illness danger. In S. Rachman (Ed.), *Contributions to medical psychology* (Vol. 2). New York: Pergamon Press.

Leventhal, H., Nerenz, D. R., & Steele, D. J. (1984). Illness representations and coping with health threats. In A. Baum, S. Taylor, & J. Singer (Eds.), *Handbook of psychology and health* (Vol. 4): *Social psychological aspects of health* (pp. 219–252). Hillsdale, NJ: Erlbaum.

Lipowski, Z. J. (1970). Physical illness, the individual and the coping process. *International Journal of Psychiatry in Medicine, 1,* 91–102.

Markus, H., & Wurf, E. (1987). The dynamic self-concept: A social psychological perspective. In M. R. Rosenzweig & L. W. Porter (Eds.), *Annual review of psychology* (Vol. 38, pp. 299–337). Palo Alto, CA: Annual Reviews.

McCaul, K. D., Thiesse-Duffy, E., & Wilson, P. (1991). Coping with medical diagnosis: The effects of at-risk versus disease labels over time. *Journal of Applied Social Psychology, 22,* 1340–1355.

Meyer, D. L., Leventhal, H., & Guttman, M. (1985). Common-sense models of illness: The example of hypertension. *Health Psychology, 4,* 115–135.

Miller, D. T., & Ross, M. (1975). Self-serving biases in attribution of causality: Fact or fiction? *Psychological Bulletin, 82,* 213–225.

Miller, S. M. (1987). Monitoring and blunting: Validation of a questionnaire to assess styles of information seeking under threat. *Journal of Personality and Social Psychology, 52,* 345–353.

Miller, S. M., Brody, D. S., & Summerton, J. (1988). Styles of coping with threat: Implications for health. *Journal of Personality and Social Psychology, 54,* 142–148.

Moore, K. A., & Ditto, P. H. (1991). *Hypochondriacal beliefs and reactions to unfavorable medical diagnoses.* Paper presented at the Annual Meeting of the American Psychological Association, San Francisco, CA.

Petersdorf, R. G., Adams, R. D., Brauwald, E., Isselbacher, K. J., Martin, J. B., & Wilson, J. D. (1983). *Harrison's principles of internal medicine* (10th ed.). New York: McGraw-Hill.

Pilowsky, I. (1967). Dimensions of hypochondriasis. *British Journal of Psychiatry, 113*, 89–93.

Pratto, F., & John, O. P. (1991). Automatic vigilance: The attention-grabbing power of negative social information. *Journal of Personality and Social Psychology, 61*, 380–391.

Prohaska, T. R., Keller, M. L., Leventhal, E. A., & Leventhal, H. (1987). Impact of symptoms and aging attribution on emotions and coping. *Health Psychology, 6*, 495–514.

Quattrone, G. A. (1985). On the congruity between internal states and action. *Psychological Bulletin, 98*, 3–40.

Rosenberg, M. (1965). *Society and the adolescent self-image.* Princeton, NJ: Princeton University Press.

Ross, L., Greene, D., & House, P. (1977). The false consensus phenomenon: An attributional bias in self-perception and social perception processes. *Journal of Experimental Social Psychology, 13*, 279–301.

Scheier, M. F., & Carver, C. S. (1985). Optimism, coping, and health: Assessment and implications of generalized outcome expectancies. *Health Psychology, 4*, 219–247.

Schuman, H., & Johnson, M. P. (1976). Attitudes and behavior. *Annual Review of Sociology, 2*, 161–207.

Schwarz, N. (1990). Feelings as information: Informational and motivational functions of affective states. In E. T. Higgins & R. M. Sorrentino (Eds.), *The handbook of motivation and cognition: Foundations of social behavior* (Vol. 2, pp. 527–561). New York: Guilford Publications, Inc.

Silverman, I. (1974). Consequences, racial discrimination, and the principle of belief congruence. *Journal of Personality and Social Psychology, 29*, 497–508.

Skelton, J. A., & Croyle, R. T. (Eds.). (1991). *Mental representation in health and illness.* New York: Springer-Verlag.

Snyder, M. (1984). When belief creates reality. In L. Berkowitz (Ed.), *Advances in experimental social psychology* (Vol. 18, pp. 248–305). New York: Academic Press.

Suls, J., & Fletcher, B. (1985). The relative efficacy of avoidant and nonavoidant coping strategies: A meta-analysis. *Health Psychology, 4*, 249–288.

Taylor, S. E. (1983). Adjustment to threatening events: A theory of cognitive adaptation. *American Psychologist, 38*, 1161–1173.

Tetlock, P. E., & Levi, A. (1982). Attribution bias: On the inconclusiveness of the cognition-motivation debate. *Journal of Experimental Social Psychology, 18*, 68–88.

Tversky, A., & Kahneman, D. (1974). Judgment under uncertainty: Heuristics and biases. *Sciences, 185*, 1124–1131.

Ullman, L. P. (1962). An empirically derived MMPI scale which measures facilitation-inhibition of recognition of threatening stimuli. *Journal of Clinical Psychology, 18*, 127–132.

Visotsky, H. M., Hamburg, D. A., Goss, M. E., & Lebovitz, B. A. (1961). Coping under extreme stress: Observations of patients with severe poliomyelitis. *Archives of General Psychiatry, 5*, 423–448.

Weinstein, N. D. (1982). Unrealistic optimism about susceptibility to health problems. *Journal of Behavioral Medicine, 5*, 441–460.

————. (1987). Unrealistic optimism about susceptibility to health problems: Conclusions from a community-wide sample. *Journal of Behavioral Medicine, 10,* 481–500.

Wicker, A. W. (1969). Attitudes vs. actions: The relationship of verbal and overt behavioral responses to attitude objects. *Journal of Social Issues, 41,* 41–78.

Zola, I. K. (1966). Culture and symptoms—An analysis of patients' presenting complaints. *American Sociological Review, 31,* 615–630.

II

Where Do We Go from Here?

8

Toward an Understanding of the Psychological Consequences of Screening

THERESA M. MARTEAU

Studies of the psychological effects of screening reveal some unexpected findings. The emotional impact of screening in high-risk groups for conditions for which no treatment is available is often less severe than expected. By contrast, high levels of distress are evident in people recalled on population-based screening programs. Attempts to reduce or keep risks low by encouraging people to alter their behavior following screening have not been very successful. That these findings have caused some surprise suggests a need to develop better models from which to understand and predict responses to receipt of information about threats to health.

The review chapters in this book illustrate the psychological themes that run through the approaches to, and results of, research on the psychological effects of a variety of health-related screening programs. This chapter will discuss some of these themes, before considering the role of psychological research in this area.

COGNITIVE AND EMOTIONAL RESPONSES

The conditions for which screening is available differ in whether they are amenable to treatment. For Huntington's disease and human immunodeficiency virus (HIV) infection, no treatments are available. Contrary to many expectations, responses of those found to be at high risk on testing for carrying the gene for Huntington's disease have not been extremely negative (Tyler, et al., 1992). For example, distress 6 months after testing was not associated with results of testing (Tibben,

185

1993). As discussed in Croyle and Lerman's chapter (Chapter 2), Wiggins and colleagues (1992) found that distress declined after testing for those who got a positive test result as well as for those who got a negative result. This is in contrast with those who were tested and for whom no result was forthcoming, whose distress was unaltered. Jemmott, Sanderson, and Miller (Chapter 5) concluded from their review of the literature that those who received the news that they were positive for HIV showed some distress after receiving their results, but this generally dissipated by around 3 weeks.

In contrast with Huntington's disease and HIV infection, there is treatment available for cervical and breast abnormalities, including cancer. Yet the psychological effects of a positive test result for cervical and breast screening are sometimes as marked as the effects of a positive result for Huntington's disease or HIV. For example, 3 months after screening, 41% of women who had a benign lesion continued to worry about breast cancer, and 25% of women suffered adverse effects upon their mood (Lerman and colleagues, 1991). Women who received positive results from routine mammography that were subsequently found to be false remained anxious 1 year later (Gram, Lund, & Slenker, 1990). Very high levels of anxiety have been found among women undergoing colposcopy examination following an abnormal cervical smear result. In one study, we found that anxiety levels were higher than those of patients the night before surgery (Marteau, Walker, Giles, & Smail, 1990). All of these women had precancerous cell changes; none had cancer.

There are several possible reasons why responses to learning of high risk for untreatable and lethal conditions, such as Huntington's disease and HIV infection, have been less negative than expected and responses to population-based screening have been more adverse than expected. These explanations include the self-selection of those undergoing testing; motivation for undergoing testing; cognitive appraisal of test results; and the ways in which screening programs are organized.

1. *Self-selection of those undergoing testing.* Only a minority, between 5% and 20% of those at risk for Huntington's disease and HIV infection, undergo testing. Of these, a small proportion are already experiencing symptoms of the disease. Those choosing not to undergo predictive testing for Huntington's disease fear more difficulty in dealing with a positive test result than those who do not undergo testing (Tibben, 1993). It is therefore possible that those who choose to undergo screening are those who are most prepared for a positive rest result. In contrast, uptake rates for population-based screening programs for risks of breast and cervical cancer are over 70%. High levels of recruit-

ment in these programs may reflect more situational influences upon uptake than decisions that encompass anticipated coping with test results (Bekker et al., 1993). It is therefore possible that many of those entering these programs have thought less about receiving a positive result than those who are at high risk and hence may be less prepared for such an outcome. Janis (1959) describes the beneficial effects of psychological preparation as facilitating the "work of worry," an important antecedent to reducing anxiety after stressful events.

2. *Uncertainty about health status.* Motivation for undergoing testing may vary in different screening programs. In population-based screening programs, people may undergo screening with the aim of confirming that they are not at risk. For those not receiving this confirmation, the results of screening may shift them from a state of certainty about their health to a state of uncertainty. By contrast, those participating in screening programs who have already been identified as being at high risk may undergo screening to reduce uncertainty. In this situation, any test result, be it positive or negative, will reduce uncertainty. Evidence to support this comes from the prospective study of the effects of testing for Huntington's disease, discussed above (Wiggins et al., 1992). Distress decreased following testing both for those who got negative results and for those who received positive test results. Distress was unchanged in those who could not be given a risk figure and hence whose risk status was unaltered. Also compatible with this explanation of different responses to high-risk and population-based screening is the differential emotional effects of false-positive results according to the prior risks of those screened. Younger pregnant women not previously identified as being at increased risk of having a child with Down's syndrome experienced greater and more sustained anxiety following a positive test result on screening for Down's syndrome than did older women, previously identified as having an increased risk (Marteau, Kidd, et al., 1988). Evidence for the aversiveness of introducing uncertainty about health status comes from several sources. In an analogue study by Cioffi (1991) (see Ditto & Croyle, Chapter 7), uncertainty about test results, in contrast with receiving a clear positive or negative result, was associated with more concern about health. Many clinically based studies report long-term distress in some of those receiving false-positive results on screening, in part explained by the experience of uncertainty (e.g., Tymstra, 1986; Lerman et al., 1991).

3. *Cognitive appraisal of results.* How people respond to information about risks to their health is sometimes influenced by a motivation to protect the self from threatening information. This is most fully ex-

plored in the laboratory-based studies of Ditto, Jemmott, and Croyle (Chapter 7). Such defensive appraisals are most likely to operate when a threat is ambiguous and serious. The operation of such processes is one explanation for the observation that those found to be HIV positive, or at high risk for developing Huntington's disease, do not necessarily experience more distress than those receiving positive results on routine breast or cervical cancer screening, which entails a lower risk of being affected for conditions which are to varying degrees treatable. One possible explanation is that for most people cancer is unambiguous as a health threat, and therefore defensive cognitive appraisals do not operate. Operational definitions of ambiguity are a necessary first step to determining its role in defensive appraisal.

4. *Pretest counseling.* Health professionals have, understandably, been very concerned about the effects of positive test results where there are few, if any, treatment options. This is reflected in the provision of detailed guidelines for mandatory counseling for testing for HIV status and Huntington's disease. In population-based screening programs, the amount and type of counseling to be provided has been less well observed. There is a general principle that people should be allowed to decide whether to participate in screening programs. There is, however, evidence to show both that pretest counseling does not take place and that it is often ineffective. Obstetricians and midwives presenting prenatal screening tests routinely provide little information (Marteau, Slack, Kidd, & Shaw, 1992; Marteau, Plenicar, & Kidd, 1993). Reflecting this, participants' knowledge of tests undergone, including whether they have been undergone at all, is frequently poor (Smith, Williams, Sibert, & Harper, 1990; Bradley, Parsons & Clarke, 1993; Marteau et al., 1988).

The better predictors of cognitive and emotional responses to screening therefore appear to be why people are tested, their states of uncertainty prior to testing, the ambiguity perceived in the test result, and pretest preparation. From this it is predicted that the most adverse reactions to a positive result will be found in those for whom undergoing screening was not the result of a personal decision about the health threat, who consider themselves to be healthy, and who undergo testing having received little, if any, pretest counseling. These are testable hypotheses. There have been several studies attempting to ameliorate adverse emotional responses to screening by intervening after results have been received. There have, however, been few controlled studies of the effects of the presentation of testing or test results to determine whether any adverse psychological effects may be prevented as opposed to just ameliorated once they have occurred. The results of one study suggest that raised anxiety may be prevented following detection of a positive result on screening by increasing the ambiguity of the result (Rudd et al., 1986). Those given their results with a reassuring message about the implications of hypertension, stressing the unreliability of blood pressure measurement, showed no change in anxiety, in contrast to those provided with a more traditional message about the risks of hypertension, who become more anxious. Whether increasing pretest uncertainty about health status or preparing people for a positive result before testing avoids raised levels of anxiety after testing awaits investigation.

BEHAVIORAL RESPONSES

People seem to make few if any changes in their behavior following screening from which they gain information about their health risks. Strecher and Kreuter (Chapter 6) find no strong evidence from randomized controlled studies of cognitive or behavioral changes following health risk assessments (HRA). Jemmott, Sanderson, and Miller, in reviewing the effects of HIV screening (Chapter 5), find little evidence for behavior change, either to reduce risks or to keep risks low.

There are several possible explanations. The first, which is suggested by Strecher and Kreuter (Chapter 6), is that health risk assessment interventions are uninformed by psychological models of behavior change. Typically, such interventions are based on a simple but invalid model of behavior in which health-related behavior is seen as determined largely by knowledge of risk. Provision of accurate information about health risks is therefore considered to lead to behavior that will reduce these risks. In contrast, social cognition and behavioral models consider knowledge just one of many factors that influence behavior. It remains to be determined whether the use of psychological models to design HRA interventions will result in the predicted behavioral changes.

Perhaps, more importantly, we need a behavioral analysis of why those organizing HRA programs, and indeed other programs attempting to alter behavior, do not routinely use psychological expertise either in designing or in executing their programs, even when evidence for its effectiveness exists. Possible reasons include the conceptualization of the problem and perceptions of psychologists. Public health specialists may hold the implicit model of behavior, described above, in which the main predictor of health-related behavior is knowledge of risks and how to alter them. Perhaps psychologists don't disseminate their findings sufficiently well into the public health arena. If this is so, then one approach to enhancing the input of psychology and hence the likely success of these programs is to provide public health specialists with more valid models of behavior. Another possible reason why psychology is infrequently used in health promotion programs is that psychologists are not primarily considered experts in behavior and behavior change. This is perhaps more likely to be the case in the United Kingdom than in North America. Research on the barriers to the involvement of psychology in these programs may help reduce the number of ineffective programs aimed at altering health-related behavior.

People's own judgments of their risks often differ from those they are given following HRA (Avis, Smith, & McKinlay, 1989; Marteau, Kinmonth, Pyke, & Thompson, in press). Some of those found to be at high risk will hold a different view of their risks and therefore see no reason to alter their behavior. A review of the literature concerning self-assessed and medically derived estimates of risks shows that self-assessed health is an independent and frequently better predictor of mortality than risks derived from HRA formulae (Idler, 1992). There are several possible explanations for this finding. Individuals may use more personally relevant information that is not gathered during routine HRA exercises. Another explanation is that judgments of health may be associated with mood, which may have an independent effect upon health status. Caution is therefore prudent before intervening to make perceptions of risk more consonant with risk estimates derived from epidemiologically based assessments.

A further factor that may impede behavioral change is the emotional effects of screening. Lerman and Rimer (Chapter 4) report the results of one of Lerman and colleagues' findings of a curvilinear relationship between breast cancer worries and breast self-examination in women following an abnormal screening result: women with moderate levels of anxiety were more likely to practice breast self-examination than women with low or high levels of anxiety.

Sometimes the emotional consequences of screening not only may fail to produce desirable behavior, but may sometimes result in behaviors that increase risk. Such an effect seemed to be evident following detection of alpha-1-antitrypsin deficiency. The objective of such screening is to protect affected children from concentrated air pollutants (mainly cigarette smoke) in the hope of preventing or postponing lung disease in adulthood. At follow-up, about half the mothers and one third of the fathers were judged by a psychiatrist to have made a poor emotional adjustment to the child's alpha-1-antitrypsin deficiency. In addition, fathers of these children smoked twice as frequently as fathers in the control group (McNeil, Sveger, & Thelin, 1988).

For those who receive a low risk result, such as with HIV testing, studies do not reveal a consistent reduction in high-risk behavior. Jemmott, Sanderson, and Miller (Chapter 5) argue that this may be due to the positive reinforcement of previous behavior: if previous behavior put an individual at risk, receiving a negative test result reinforces previous behavior, perhaps encouraging a false sense of invulnerability. Tymstra and Bieleman (1987), in a study of risk factors screening for coronary heart disease, described this phenomenon as the "certificate of health effect" that follows from a low risk result on screening. A study of the behavioral effects of a negative breast biopsy by Haefner, Becker, Janz, & Rott (1989), reported by Lerman and Rimer (Chapter 4), found that the consequences of a negative result seemed to depend upon previous health-related behavior. The extent to which women had engaged in breast self-examination before receiving a negative result on a breast biopsy predicted their subsequent behavior. Contrary to the positive reinforcement hypothesis, women who had not practiced regular breast self-examination were more likely to do so after their negative results. In contrast, those who had practiced regular breast self-examination were less likely to do so after a negative biopsy result. Documenting the cognitive mediators of these behavioral consequences of negative results on screening may resolve the apparent inconsistencies across studies.

RESEARCH APPROACHES

The limitations of studies to date in this area observed by the authors in this book are those found in any body of psychological research. They concern study designs, measures, and theoretical underpinnings.

Study Designs

Three distinct sets of research approaches are discernible in this area: clinical descriptive studies, clinical studies using experimental designs, and laboratory-based experimental designs. The first are most numerous. The most valuable data, however, are likely to be those obtained from experimental designs and from prospective, rather than retrospective, studies. Experimental designs, however, are not always feasible or appropriate. Although, for example, it may not be appropriate to randomly allocate people to screening, it can be appropriate to randomly allocate people to the offer of screening, or the manner in which screening is offered. This was the design used in a study reported by Jemmott, Sanderson, and Miller (Chapter 5), in which men attending a clinic for sexually transmitted diseases were randomly allocated to the offer of HIV testing or to information about free HIV testing sites (Wenger, Linn, Epstein, & Shapiro, 1991).

Laboratory-based experimental designs have proved a rich source of information about the psychological processes influencing responses to screening. But as well as recognizing the strengths of this paradigm, its limitations must also be recognized, as discussed by Ditto and Croyle (Chapter 7). Laboratory studies are based on diagnoses, hypothetical and real, of limited severity. Participants in such studies have hitherto been young, healthy university students. Perhaps more importantly, undergoing screening in a laboratory does not simulate the different pathways that those undergoing screening in clinics might follow. If, as suggested by some clinical studies, the decision to undergo screening prepares and hence predicts responses to screening in clinical settings, this effect will not be apparent in laboratory studies as currently designed.

Problems of generalizability of findings are also presented by many clinical studies. Clinical descriptive studies, for example, rarely involve more than one center or more than one team of health professionals. This is infrequently acknowledged in discussions of results. Hence outcomes are attributed to the event of interest: a test result. It is likely, however, that responses will be influenced by a variety of factors of which the test result is just one. Failure to acknowledge the situational influences upon responses may be one explanation for apparent inconsistencies in the literature on the effects of screening. For example, receiving a low risk result on screening for risk of heart disease is sometimes associated with raised level of anxiety (Stoate, 1989) and at other times, with reduced levels of anxiety (Tymstra & Bieleman, 1987). It is possible that these different effects are due to differences in how participants are recruited for screening, as well as differences in the information they were given before and after testing. Because many studies involve just one screening program, they do not allow examination of the effect of the organization of the screening program upon responses. The organization of programs needs to be incorporated into study designs to determine its relative effect.

Measures

As several authors in this book point out, comparability of responses across studies is sometimes hampered by the use of different and sometimes unstandardized measures. There is, however, a fair degree of overlap in the measures used to assess mood, with the Impact of Events scale (Horowitz, Wilner, & Alvarez, 1979), Spielberger State Anxiety Inventory (Spielberger, Gorsuch, & Lushene, 1970), and the Beck Depression Inventory (Beck, Ward, Mendelson, Mock & Erbaugh, 1961) among the most frequently used. Standardized measures of behavior, however, are more difficult to obtain. Reliance on self-report measures, for example in assessing sexual behavior, may severely compromise the validity of any results. More research effort needs to be directed toward evaluating different methods of obtaining valid data. One approach to this has been to compare responses obtained through questionnaires with those obtained using in-depth interviews (Wight, in press).

As well as considering the type of measure to be used to assess a particular variable, the evaluation of outcomes and their inter-relationships also need to be considered. Raised anxiety or defensively optimistic assessments of a threat are sometimes deemed inappropriate, and hence suitable targets for intervention, as discussed by Lerman and Rimer (Chapter 4) and Ditto and Croyle (Chapter 7). Ditto and Croyle, for example, present evidence that points to the functional independence of cognitive appraisals and behavior. Lerman and Rimer present evidence that points to the value of a certain amount of anxiety as a precursor to health-protective behavior. It is clear that the consequences of these cognitive and emotional outcomes need to be considered in relation to each other as well as in relation to overt behavior before attempts are made to alter any of them. The timing of measurements is also important (Turnquist, Harvey, & Anderson, 1988): psychological outcomes are usually most appropriately seen within a wider context of adaptation or coping over time. So, for example, high anxiety at one point may herald more rapid adjustment than lower levels of anxiety.

Theoretical Approaches

All the contributors are critical of the literature for failing to use more explicitly one or more of the many possible psychological theories available either to generate research questions or to explain findings. A simple stimulus-response model is frequently implicit in clinically based studies assessing the effects of screening. The stimulus is the test result; the main analysis involves comparison between those receiving negative and those receiving positive test results. The limitations of this approach are evident when test results are found to be weak or insignificant predictors of responses (e.g., Tibben, 1993). Relatively little attention has been paid to psychological processes that may mediate or moderate the relationship between testing and responses in clinically based studies. There is also a tendency for studies to be reported without reference to any context, such as how screening was conducted or how the test results were presented. As discussed in several chapters, relatively little attention has been paid to the social context, particularly the family and social support systems of those tested. Recent research findings on the effects of Huntington's disease suggest that the responses of the partner has an important bearing on the response of the individual tested. In a study of women undergoing prenatal screening for neural tube defects, those with high social support were least distressed following a positive test result (Robinson, Hibbard, & Laurence, 1984). Croyle and Lerman (Chapter 2) comment on the paucity of studies that have addressed the responses of different ethnic groups to screening. The lack of such data is one factor that lies behind differences in opinion in how to offer prenatal screening for fetal abnormalities to women of Pakistani origin in the United Kingdom. This follows publication of a recent study documenting high risk of congenital abnormality, resulting from first-cousin marriages, which is common in this community (Bundey & Alam, 1993). Some data on how these communities view first- or second-cousin marriage, inheritance, prenatal screening, abortion, and disability is a necessary first step in planning appropriate screening services.

While context may affect individual responses to screening, screening itself may be affecting some aspects of this context. There has been a tendency to consider the effects of screening only among those undergoing screening and, occasionally, their families. It is possible, however, that the mere availability of screening may affect the way in which health and illness are perceived by the population, including attributions for the causes of illness (Duster, 1990; Lippman, 1991). Evidence to support this comes from an analogue study in which doctors and nurses were found to hold more negative attitudes toward patients who had not followed recommended health actions, which included screening, in contrast with their more positive attitudes toward patients with the same condition who had followed relevant health actions (Marteau & Riordan, 1992). In a similarly designed study involving health professionals, patients, and the general public in three European countries, women who rejected the offer of prenatal testing were seen as more responsible and more to blame for having a child with Down's syndrome than women who also had an affected child but had not been offered the test (Marteau & Drake, in press).

These analogue studies represent just one approach to examining the wider social implications of screening. Using models that incorporate social context in explaining behaviors (Winnett, 1985) provides a broader range of research questions than those arising from the immediate clinical perspective.

ROLES FOR PSYCHOLOGY IN SCREENING RESEARCH

The study of health-related screening will be one of the most prolific areas for health psychologists in the coming years, given the increasing emphasis in Western health care upon disease prevention, coupled with rapid developments in biomedicine, particularly those arising from human genome analysis. It is therefore pertinent to consider the role of psychological research in this area. Several current roles are discernible, encompassing the description, explanation, and changing of patients' behavior and, less frequently, that of health professionals.

1. *Describing the effects of screening.* Psychologists are increasingly involved in evaluating screening programs, most often in descriptive studies. As discussed above, the use of experimental designs in evaluating programs will further understanding of both psychological processes and how best to offer screening in order to enhance benefits and to reduce or avoid adverse effects. Descriptive studies could usefully be extended to consider the impact of testing not just on individuals, but also their families, health professionals, and different social and ethnic groups, as well as health care planners.

2. *Determining effective and efficient organization of screening programs.* Increasingly, psychologists are involved in the early evaluative stages of screening programs. In organizing and evaluating any program, it is first necessary to determine the goals of the program. These are not always articulated. If, for example, the goal of HRA is to enhance health, broadly defined to include psychological health, then the incorporation of psychological outcome measures in any assessment of such screening is essential. If the primary goal of prenatal screening is to reduce the birth incidence of certain abnormalities, then such tests should be presented in such a way as to maximize uptake. If the primary goal is to facilitate informed decision making in the face of reproductive risks, then screening should be set up to maximize parental understanding of tests and any test results, and the evaluation should be in terms of quality of decision making, not numbers of affected pregnancies terminated. Although these goals are not necessarily in conflict, evidence suggests that achieving the latter (good decision making) compromises achievement of the former (high uptake). A further empirical question is: who decides what the goals of screening are? Having articulated the goals of screening, controlled

studies can then be set up to determine how these are achieved most effectively and efficiently.

3. *Changing behavior*. Psychologists may also be involved in screening programs that involve attempts to change people's behavior to reduce or avoid health risks. There are two possible pitfalls with this role. First, the evidence for the benefits of intervening are not always established. Given the history of medicine (Skrabenek & McCormick, 1989), it is perhaps important that psychologists maintain an intellectually skeptical approach to medical activity. Second, there are too few psychologists available for involvement in every program. In the United States, for example, Strecher and Kreuter (Chapter 6) report that as many as 30% of worksites use some form of HRA. Given the discrepancy between the size of the problem and the number of psychologists, psychological input would be better restricted to the development and evaluation of interventions that can then be conducted by health professionals trained in behavioral techniques.

4. *Determining the provision of screening services*. The setting up of a screening program is the result of a decision and as such falls within the domain of psychological study. Hitherto, there has been little psychological research on the factors that determine the implementation and resourcing of some prevention services and not others. Such decisions may be influenced by several considerations, of which effectiveness at reducing morbidity or mortality is just one. Other influential factors are the nature of the health problem, the attributions about its causes, and the economic incentives of those who develop screening tests. The attributional model of helping behavior predicts that people are more likely to offer assistance if the cause of the problem is seen as uncontrollable (Weiner, 1980). There is some evidence that this model is useful in predicting the behavior of health professionals as well as others (Brewin, 1984; Marteau & Riordan, 1992). This may therefore be one factor explaining the greater enthusiasm for screening and intervention for those at risk for inherited diseases than for those at risk for smoking-related diseases. Some screening programs may be driven more by technology availability (such as carrier testing for cystic fibrosis following the isolation of the gene) than by greatest health need (such as low-birthweight babies born to socially and economically disadvantaged women).

Aside from describing how decisions about the provision of screening services are to be made, evidence from psychological studies can be used to inform debates about whether a screening program should be set up at all. Such evidence might include the advantages and disadvantages of screening programs as perceived by clinicians and public health specialists, as well as those eligible to undergo screening.

All are possible roles for health psychologists. Psychologists need to work to frame questions about the psychological effects of screening and not just devote their energies to addressing the questions raised by those who organize screening services.

CONCLUSION

There is now a substantial body of research on the psychological impact of screening for disease prevention and detection. This work provides a good basis from which to develop the next generation of studies. Two developments to be encouraged are the use of experimental designs, particularly in clinical settings, and the use of psychological models to explain and predict responses to screening. Given the amount of activity in this area, theoretical developments and practical applications of psychology are likely to be very great over the next few years.

ACKNOWLEDGMENTS

This manuscript was prepared while the author was supported by a grant from The Wellcome Trust, United Kingdom.

REFERENCES

Avis, N. E., Smith, K. W., & McKinlay, J. B. (1989). Accuracy of perceptions of heart attack risk: What influences perceptions and can they be changed? *American Journal of Public Health, 79,* 1608–1612.

Beck, A. T., Ward, C. H., Mendelson, M., Mock, J. E., & Erbaugh, J. (1961). An inventory for measuring depression. *Archives of General Psychiatry, 4,* 561–571.

Bekker, H., Modell, M., Denniss, G., Mathew, C., Silver, A., Bobrow, M., & Marteau, T. M. (1993). Uptake of cystic fibrosis testing in primary care: supply push or demand pull? *British Medical Journal, 306,* 1584–1586.

Bradley, D. M., Parsons, E. P., & Clarke, A. J. (1993). Experience with screening newborns for Duchenne muscular dystrophy in Wales. *British Medical Journal 306,* 357–360.

Brewin, C. (1984). Perceived controllability of life-events and willingness to prescribe psychotropic drugs. *British Journal of Social Psychology, 23,* 285–287.

Bundey, S., & Alam, A. (1993). A five year prospective study of the health of children in different ethnic groups with particular reference to the effect of in-breeding. *European Journal of Human Genetics, 1,* 206–219.

Cioffi, D. (1991). Asymmetry of doubt in medical self-diagnosis: The ambiguity of "uncertain wellness." *Journal of Personality and Social Psychology, 61,* 969–980.

Duster, T. C. (1990). *Backdoor to eugenics.* New York: Routledge, Chapman and Hall.

Gram, I. T., Lund, E., & Slenker, S. E. (1990). Quality of life following a false positive mammogram. *British Journal of Cancer, 62,* 1018–1022.

Haefner, D. P., Becker, M. H., Janz, N. K., & Rutt, W. M. (1989). Impact of a negative breast biopsy on subsequent breast self-examination practice. *Patient Education and Counselling, 14,* 137–146.

Horowitz, M., Wilner, N., & Alvarez, W. (1979). Impact of Events Scale: A measure of subjective stress. *Psychosomatic Medicine, 41*(3), 209–218.

Idler, E. L. (1992). Self-assessed health and mortality: A review of studies. In S. Maes, H. Leventhal, & M. Johnston, (Eds.), *International review of Health Psychology,* (pp. 33–54) John Wiley & Sons Ltd.

Janis, I. L. (1959). *Psychological stress.* New York: John Wiley & Sons, Inc.

Lerman, C., Trock, B., Rimer, B., Boyce, A., Jepson, C., Engstrom, P. (1991). Psychological and behavioral implications of abnormal mammograms. *Annals of Internal Medicine, 114,* 657–661.

Lippman, A. (1991). Prenatal genetic testing and screening: Constructing needs and reinforcing inequities. *American Journal of Law and Medicine, 17,* 15–50.

Marteau, T. M., & Drake, H. (in press). Attributions for disability: The influence of genetic screening. *Social Science & Medicine.*

Marteau, T. M., Kidd, J., Cook, R., Johnston, M., Michie, S., Shaw, R.W., & Slack, J. (1988). Screening for Down's syndrome [Letter] *British Medical Journal, 297,* 1469.

Marteau, T. M., Johnston, M., Plenicar, M., Shaw, R. W., & Slack, J. (1988). Development of a self-administered questionnaire to measure women's knowledge of prenatal screening and diagnostic tests. *Journal of Psychosomatic Research, 32,* 403–408.

Marteau, T. M., Kinmonth, A. L., Pyke, S., & Thompson, S. (in press). Readiness for life-style advice: perceptions of risk prior to screening. *British Journal of General Practice.*

Marteau, T. M., Plenicar, M., & Kidd, J. (1993). Obstetricians presenting amniocentesis to pregnant women: Practice observed. *Journal of Reproductive and Infant Psychology, 11,* 3–10.

Marteau, T. M., & Riordan, D. C. (1992). Staff attitudes to patients: The influence of causal attributions for illness. *British Journal of Clinical Psychology, 31,* 107–110.

Marteau, T. M., Slack, J., Kidd, J., & Shaw, R. W. (1992). Presenting a routine screening test in antenatal care: Practice observed. *Public Health, 106,* 131–141.

Marteau, T. M., Walker, P., Giles, J., & Smail, M. (1990). Anxiety and coping in women undergoing colposcopy following abnormal cervical smears. *British Journal of Obstetric Gynecology, 97,* 859–61.

McNeil, T. F., Sveger, T., Thelin, T. (1988). Psychosocial effects of screening for somatic risk: the Swedish alpha-1-antitripsin experience. *Thorax, 43,* 505–507.

Robinson, J., Hibbard, B. M., & Laurence, K. M. (1984). Anxiety during a crisis: Emotional effects of screening for neural tube defects. *Journal of Psychosomatic Research, 28:* 163–169.

Rudd, P., Price, M. G., Graham, L. E., Beilstein, B. A., Tarbell, S. J. H., Bacchetti, P., & Fortmann, S. P. (1986). Consequences of worksite hypertension screening. *American Journal of Medicine, 80,* 853–860.

Skrabenek, P., & Mccormick, J. (1989). *Follies and fallacies in medicine.* Glasgow: Tarragan Press.

Smith, R. A., Williams, D. K., Sibert, J. R., & Harper, P. S. (1990). Attitudes of mothers to neonatal screening for Duchenne muscular dystrophy. *British Medical Journal, 300,* 1112.

Spielberger, C. D., Gorsuch, R. L., & Lushene, R. E. (1970). Manual for the State-Trait Anxiety Inventory. Palo Alto: Consulting Psychologists Press, Inc.

Stoate, H. (1989). Can health screening damage your health? *Journal of the Royal College of General Practitioners, 39,* 193–195.

Tibben, A. (1993). *What is knowledge but grieving? On psychological effects of presymptomatic DNA-testing for Huntington's disease.* Thesis presented in Rotterdam.

Turnquist, D. C., Harvey, J. H., & Anderson, B. L. (1988). Attributions and adjustment to life-threatening illness. *British Journal of Clinical Psychology, 27,* 55–65.

Tyler, A., Morris, M., Lazarou, L., Meredith, L., Myring, J., & Harper, P. (1992). Presymptomatic testing for Huntington's disease in Wales 1987–90. *British Journal of Psychiatry, 161,* 481–488.

Tymstra, T. (1986). False positive results in screening tests: experience of parents of children screened for congenital hypothyroidism. *Family Practice 3,* 92–96.

Tymstra, T., & Bieleman, B. (1987). The psychosocial impact of mass screening for cardiovascular risk factors. *Family Practice, 4,* 287–290.

Weiner, B. (1980). A cognitive (attribution)-emotion-action model of motivated behavior: An analysis of judgements of help-giving. *Journal of Personality and Social Psychology, 39,* 186–200.

Wenger, N. S., Linn, L. S., Epstein, M., & Shapiro, M. F. (1991). Reduction of high-risk sexual behavior among heterosexuals undergoing HIV antibody testing: A randomized clinical trial. *American Journal of Public Health, 81,* 1580–1585.

Wiggins, S., Whyte, P., Huggins, M., Adam, S., Theilmann, J., Bloch, M., Sheps, S. B., Schechter, M. T., & Hayden, M. R. (1992). The psychological consequences of predictive testing for Huntington's disease. *The New England Journal of Medicine, 327,* 1401–1405.

Wight, D. (in press). Boy's thoughts and talk about sex in a working class locality of Glasgow. *Sociological Review.*

Winnett, R. A. (1985). Ecobehavioral assessment in health life-styles: Concepts and methods. In P. Karoly (Ed.), *Measurement strategies in health psychology* (pp. 147–181). New York: Wiley.

9

Screening for Disease Detection and Prevention: Some Comments and Future Perspectives

TORBJØRN MOUM

Testing for disease and health risk today is done on a routine basis in all industrialized nations. Tests for diabetes, hypertension, urinary tract infection, and other disorders are most commonly performed on individuals in a doctor-patient relationship. The term *screening*, however, usually refers to large-scale testing that is organized as a program aimed at a defined population. Quite often such programs are carried out under public auspices.

Whether the detection of disease and health risk is most efficiently carried out through the screening of entire populations or through the ongoing relationship between patient and doctor obviously depends on the condition in question. However, many of the ethical dilemmas and public health implications of testing asymptomatic individuals are the same regardless of the exact organizational context in which testing takes place (for a slightly different view, see Gochfeld, 1992).

If there are documented—or highly probable—negative psychosocial effects of screening for disease prevention and detection, these could influence our decisions about (1) the type of disease or condition for which screening should occur, (2) what type of subjects or patients should be screened, and (3) the way in which given screening operations are carried out and followed up. The chapters of the present volume have focused almost exclusively on the *individual-level* sequelae of being a screenee, with more of an emphasis on the "psycho"

200

than the "social" of psychosocial effects. I shall also offer some comments on the screening impact as experienced by the individual screenee. However, there are several other issues pertaining specifically to the *societal* effects of carrying out large-scale screening that need to be considered. These are effects that do not necessarily have an impact on screening participants or their immediate family, but which may nevertheless be of concern to those planning and carrying out screening operations.

INDIVIDUAL-LEVEL EFFECT

Psychological Distress

A major focus in the literature to date has been on the psychological distress or reduced quality of life experienced by screenees who are "labeled" by receiving a medical diagnosis or negative information regarding their health risk factors. This type of research interest obviously draws on the kind of reasoning that also underlies the quality-adjusted life years (QUALY) approach in prioritizing in health care generally: There appears to be a need for keeping some sort of a ledger in which the gain in longevity *times* the life quality of the life-years gained is weighed against the cost of administering the health care required for a given disease or condition. In the present context the argument would be that if—in addition to the economic cost of carrying out the screening in the first place—the quality of the remaining life-years of screenees (and not only the true positives) is extremely negatively affected by the screening process, there must be a point at which we consider letting nature take its course. This is of course a particularly pertinent issue for conditions for which there is no cure (in the present volume, Huntington's disease, AIDS, and cystic fibrosis are frequently cited examples).

With diseases for which there is a cure or at least a partial cure, severely reduced quality of life among previously undiagnosed individuals could induce us to wait for the disease/condition to become symptomatic and simply incur the cost of caring for those cases that theoretically could have been ameliorated or prevented by carrying out a screening. Similarly, with recognized risk factors that may be modified (such as blood pressure and cholesterol) the longevity gained among true-positive screenees who are successfully treated is only part of the equation. What if all of their remaining life-years are far less enjoyable than a shorter—but happier—life span had the condition not been detected? Further, what if there is a very considerable proportion of screenees that are treated and put on medication, and that experience the same deterioration in life quality, yet whose health and longevity *never* would have been negatively affected by the risk factor if no treatment had been instituted (since we are talking only about risk)?

The QUALY reasoning at least partly implicit in monitoring levels of psychological distress among screenees clearly speaks to such issues. It is interesting, therefore, to observe what surprisingly attenuated (long-term) effects on psychological distress are found by most of the research reviewed in the present volume. According to Jemmott, Sanderson, and Miller (Chapter 5), even people who learn that they are HIV seropositive react with only a transient (albeit substantial) increase in psychological distress. The same appears to be true of people who are informed of abnormal genetic test results (Croyle & Lerman, Chapter 2) or of being exposed to carcinogens (Lerman & Rimer, Chapter 4). Information about more "benign" conditions and risk factors such as elevated blood pressure and cholesterol levels sometimes even appear to result in *improved* subjective well-being among those diagnosed (Mann, 1984; Havas et al., 1991; the latter cited by Glanz & Gilboy, Chapter 3). Do these findings indicate that most people have an uncanny capacity to deal with (the threat of) disease or a drastically reduced life expectancy or should we look for a flaw in the data?

The most important caveats to be invoked with respect to the apparent lack of long-term increases in psychological distress among screening positives have already been pointed out in the various chapters of this volume: (1) People who choose to be tested are by definition, self-selected and may in part be psychologically and behaviorally prepared for dealing with the bad news. Investigating whether self-selection is a significant factor is hard, however, since randomly assigning screening participation (or information about results) usually is not practically possible or indeed ethically justifiable. (2) Most of the scales used to measure a reduction in life quality or subjective well-being are very *global* and may not capture the finer details of worry over illness, symptom awareness, and less favorable self-evaluations of health.

In addition one should consider the possibility that the rating scale items querying respondents about their level of subjective well-being somehow contain a built-in bias toward "regression to the mean." When one questions respondents about the intensity and/or duration of certain feeling states—typically with an explicit time frame referring to the last week or two—there is reason to believe that most people would tend to report not only the "absolute" level or frequency of those feeling states, but to a considerable extent *deviations* from their own typical mean. If worrying about impending disease and death does in fact permanently lower a person's average level of subjective well-being (cardinal utility *sensu stricto)*, it is still conceivable that the run-of-the-mill rating scales for anxiety, depression, and psychological distress would not be very sensitive to such changes on a long-term basis. The bulk of the variance in the items *could* be produced by relatively short-lived oscillations around the individual's personal, medium-term (e.g., postdiagnosis) average. Indeed, some rating scales for psychological distress (e.g., Goldberg's [1972] General Health Questionnaire) explicitly invite such mental relative-to-own-mean calculations to be carried out by using response categories like "more than usual," "less than usual," etc.

It would be somewhat rash to write off all zero-findings as being due to measurement artifacts, however. We know from a host of studies that people suffering from illness and impairment consistently report lower levels of psychological well-being than healthy controls (Okun, Stock, Haring, & Witter, 1984; George & Landerman, 1984). Although most results are based on cross-sectional correlations, prospective and longitudinal studies indicate that the direction of causation primarily is from morbidity to psychological distress and not vice versa (Aneshensel, Frerichs, & Huba, 1984; Kaplan, Roberts, Camacho, & Coyne, 1987). It seems reasonable to conclude, therefore, that so long as a condition remains asymptomatic, people being informed of impending disease or health risk factors to a considerable extent are able to regain their previous peace of mind, probably through such processes of denial, optimistic biases, etc. that have been described and documented in this volume. This of course does not necessarily imply that "all is well" in the field of screening for disease detection and prevention. There may be other—perhaps more indirect and long-term—costs incurred by screening participants and society at large that are equally important.

Employment and Insurance

Some of the individual-level effects of having disease or health risk factors uncovered by a medical screening that have not been specifically focused upon in this volume include employment opportunities and the availability of reasonable health, life, and disability insurance policies. A screenee who has been informed of an asymptomatic disease or a serious health risk factor cannot in good faith conceal such facts from a prospective employer or an insurer (Billings et al., 1992). Thus, being a screening positive may be a mixed blessing indeed. The screenee need not even be affected directly himself to encounter insurance and employment problems because of screening test results. Just being a *carrier* of an autosomal recessive gene (e.g., for sickle cell disease) and thus at risk for producing *sick offspring* could put health insurers (or small self-insured employers) in jeopardy of incurring higher costs. Indeed, in the case of sickle cell disease, implementing screening for the trait has affected not only screenees, but all members of the black community: because the sickle cell trait is much more prevalent among blacks, discrimination based on race alone easily may follow. According to Murray (1991) ". . . testing for sickle cell anemia followed by exclusion of those with the trait would effectively exclude one of every eight black job candidates in the U.S." (p. 57). Clearly, such prospects raise the issue of what kinds of questions insurers and employers should be allowed to ask, who has legitimate access to screening test results, and so on (also see below).

Making sure that whatever information is made available is actually fully understood and put to the right use in itself is no mean task. For example, in the case of sickle cell disease—where the controversy over screening now has raged for more than 2 decades—there are numerous documented cases of confusion regarding the nature of the disease (e.g., the assumption made by some that it is communicable), the distinction between being a carrier (having the trait) and having the disease itself, the probabilities and risks involved in a reproductive context, as well as the impact of the trait on life expectancy. As a consequence, insurance companies, employers, and official agencies (schools, the army) have been known to discriminate against individuals with sickle cell trait, usually with little grounding in medical facts (Fost, 1992).

There is little reason to believe that confusion regarding probabilities and risks will be easier to avoid with the advent of technologies that can make available to the individual a record of his or her particular genome, including mutations, and the benefits and risks of testing for the associated disorders. The sheer amount of information and the need among insurers and employers to work out some relatively simple decision rules clearly could result in very unfortunate handling of individual cases. The corporate wish to reduce the risk of future losses may take a heavy toll among individual clients and employees.

SOCIETAL-LEVEL EFFECTS

Economic Considerations

The reduction in morbidity and mortality that is the main intended result from early detection and treatment of disease or health risk factors of course always comes at a price. The economic costs of screening operations have been a major focus in cost-benefit and cost-effectiveness analyses. Considerations of pain, discomfort, and worry aside, for several risk factors or conditions it is usually possible to estimate quite accurately the economic costs of prolonging life by 1 year if one carries out a screening and starts early treatment of the screening positives. Certain of these cost-effectiveness analyses can be thought provoking because there are types of screenings and interventions that look well founded on the face of them but on closer scrutiny turn out to be extremely expensive. Thus Hulley et al. (1993) estimate that, in the general adult population, cholesterol intervention (using a cholesterol-lowering agent, lovastatin) aimed at preventing coronary disease would cost between $1 million and $10 million per year of life prolonged for women aged 25 to 44 years or men aged 25 to 34 years. They also point out that $1 million per life-year is ". . . more than 100 times the cost of other preventive interventions such as those directed at smoking or of high-technology treatments such as left main coronary bypass surgery" (p. 1417).

Cost-benefit analyses for prenatal mass screening programs for a genetic defect such as cystic fibrosis also are rather discouraging, because (1) the low sensitivity of current tests, (2) the relatively high cost of the tests themselves (in particular if several mutations are tested for in order to increase sensitivity), and (3) the enormous costs of the genetic counseling and public education programs that would be necessary together seem to add up to a prohibitive price tag (Natowicz & Alper, 1991). One could retort, purely within an economic frame of reference, that preventing the birth of patients with cystic fibrosis would cut medical expenses dramatically on a long-term basis. However, it has been estimated that more than $1 million is needed to avoid one cystic fibrosis birth, and this is approximately five times as much as the economic costs of medical care for an individual with cystic fibrosis (Wilfond & Fost, 1990). Screening *newborns* for cystic fibrosis of course only works to boost the cost of caring for such patients and at present there seem to be few if any pulmonary benefits to be reaped from early, presymptomatic treatment (Farrell & Mischler, 1992).

Despite such considerations there has been a substantial impetus for both prenatal and neonatal mass screening for cystic fibrosis. It does not seem far-fetched to tie much of the advocacy for population screening for cystic fibrosis to the enormous financial interests of the companies that would provide the diagnostic testing. Wilfond and Fost (1990) have estimated that the discovery of the gene(s) for cystic fibrosis created an immediate potential market of more than $1 billion. At least in the United States, there is today a rather close financial involvement of physicians and scientists with the commercial genetic (and other) laboratories. This fact further underscores the necessity of scrutinizing the scientific and professional validity of calls for mass screening programs generally. Financing many of the programs that have been suggested certainly would not help contain spiraling medical expenses. From the point of view of the general public (who in the final analysis is going to foot the bill), the sheer economic burden should be considered part of the direct and indirect social impact of screening programs when risks, costs, and benefits are tallied.

Insurance and Employment

It was pointed out above that individuals being tested in screening programs may encounter subsequent problems regarding employment and insurance. A natural first reaction to prevent such calamities could be to bar insurers and employers from obtaining information about screening test results. Indeed a number of regulations and guidelines already exist regarding who should be informed, confidentiality, who may access the files with information about test results, and other restrictions. Rules may vary from one state to the other. However, not only individuals may suffer from the information made available through screening for disease detection and prevention. Insurance companies and employers that do not or are not allowed to obtain medical screening information may lose their competitive edge. In the insurance industry in particular there is considerable concern that screenees may misrepresent or fail to disclose information necessary for accurate risk assessment and calculation of premiums. At the same time one suspects that persons who have received unfavorable news about their health risk status may be particularly prone to purchasing or continuing insurance (so-called adverse selection). The net result would be that insurance companies are forced to increase premiums to cover their losses, maybe to a point where low-risk individuals are induced to buy insurance elsewhere or leave the insurance market altogether (Ostrer et al., 1993). Even though insurance market dissolution and company insolvency perhaps are not very likely in the short term, the fact remains that increasingly accurate information about health risk status in the future may work to undermine the entire premise of protecting against unexpected health problems through insurance. Ironically, those who stand to lose from increased premiums and a general weakening of the insurance industry are precisely those who from a medical point of view should benefit the most from mass screening programs.

Let us assume that screening for certain conditions becomes very widespread and that—in order to make risk assessment more accurate—insurance companies are allowed to make use of any information obtained from medical screening operations. The occasional insurance applicant *without* any screening results to show for himself in such a situation may in fact come under considerable pressure to undergo testing. The insurance company would stand to gain by getting better data for setting a price and the applicant would probably hope to receive a favorable test result and a relatively reasonable insurance premium. However, for the entire pool of insured individuals, nothing much appears to have been gained (*particularly* if there is no cure for the condition for which testing occurs): (1) time and money have been spent to test individuals who really were not interested in being tested; (2) certain individuals with poor test results may be turned down by the company or discouraged by the expensive premium for high-risk individuals, in effect leaving those who have the highest probability of future need without coverage; and (3) time and money have been used by the insurance companies on a risk classification process, the net result of which, in general, will be only a *differentiation* of the premiums. If instead all applicants had been treated as a group of homogeneous exposures and everybody had paid the same premium (which is entirely feasible with the conditions for which screening occurs), less resources would have been used all around on medical tests and on collecting and processing the data necessary for risk classification. And those with the bleakest health prospects would have stood a better chance of ending up among the insured. However, to implement such a policy without creating market imbalances it is of course necessary for all insurance companies to comply.

For small self-insured employers the situation is obviously entirely different from that of large insurance companies or corporations. Small self-insured employers cannot afford to calculate in large numbers because hiring one or two employees with an asymptomatic health problem could be a financial time bomb. Hedging against future burdens by insisting that screening results be released or revealed prior to employment is quite understandable. If mandatory or near-universal screening has been instituted, there is little that individual prospective employees can do on their own to resist passing on the relevant information (or to get tested if this has not already occurred).

In the wake of the Human Genome Project, it is highly likely that new technologies will become available that will allow for fast and affordable ways of mapping, with increasing precision, any given individual's risk of disease, susceptibility to specific workplace toxins, etc. Again there would be a financial incentive for insurers and employers to utilize such technologies at their own discretion and to carry out testing even on clients or employees who express no personal interest.

The point in drawing up the above scenarios has been to show how an increased supply (or potential supply) of information about the morbidity and health risk status of a given population may trigger a demand for even more testing to be performed, perhaps with little or no medical justification. Exactly how widespread screening must be to get such processes off the ground is hard to predict. Maybe the critical mass is not defined by the proportion of the populace that is being tested for any given condition, but rather by the prevalence of screening and testing generally in society.

Medicalization

The notion that most diseases are preventable or curable appears to be embraced by more and more people, not least in the United States. Historically there is of course considerable substance to the contention that the medical profession of today has effective treatments or preventive measures for far more of the serious diseases than some decades ago (Beeson, 1980). However, health as a community value and a personal goal seems to have taken on a centrality quite out of proportion with ongoing medical progress. Some theorists have likened the growth in health awareness and the adoption of (presumed) healthy lifestyles with the advent of a new religion, where medicine is "the social guardian of morality" (Turner, 1984). In any case there is reason to believe that society's increased focus on disease and illness and the commercialization of health have fostered a public that is less satisfied with its health, more prone to seek medical attention even for minor ailments, and more intimidated by the prospect of experiencing ill health and threats to longevity than ever before (Barsky, 1988).

Screening for disease prevention and detection only works to strengthen the expectation that modern medicine coupled with a healthy lifestyle is an almost foolproof guarantee against future health problems. The clinical approach of the medical screening that some critics (e.g., Rose, 1990) claim contribute to the "medicalization of prevention" thus may have the additional unfortunate consequence of inducing a sense of failure, shame, and guilt among those individuals who are nevertheless taken ill with exactly the kind of diseases or conditions they had set out to prevent. This is indeed very relevant in connection with prenatal screening, where the broad range of technologies presently available for the early detection of congenital abnormalities easily may foster an illusion of the "perfect child" (Tymstra, 1991). For parents who are nevertheless left with a less-than-perfect child on their hands, self-blame and social stigma may result (Kielstein & Sass, 1992). Avoiding such processes of "blaming the victim" and of generating a state of generalized hypochondriasis in a population that is overwhelmingly in very good health is one of the big challenges for those planning, promoting, and following up medical screening operations.

Community Norms, Values, and Principles

Whereas screening would tend to reinforce health as a community value, there are other principles and values that could be threatened. In terms of legal liability, the counseling of screening participants derives from the same principles of *malpractice, informed consent,* and *confidentiality* that apply to other types of medical procedures (Waltz & Thigpen, 1973). In the context of mass screening operations, perhaps the most problematic of these is *informed consent* and *confidentiality*. Even though relatively few workplace genetic screening programs have been implemented, there are already several examples of suits calling for the improper disclosure of confidential medical data to a current or potential employer or to other third parties such as spouses, insurance companies, and the government (Andrews & Jaeger, 1991). With the complexity of the issues involved in genetic screening, the safeguarding of the principle of informed consent already represents a formidable task. Even with a relatively simple screening program, like that for Tay-Sachs disease, it was deemed necessary to feature extensive education to participants before screening was offered (Childs, Gordis, Kaback, & Kazazian, 1976). Other testing taking place today is considerably more involved. For example, the testing period for Huntington's disease can last up to 2 years (Terrenoire, 1992). With the extremely complex information that will be made available with the new technologies spurred by the Human Genome Project, it is indeed hard to see how one can live up to traditional notions of informed consent. As Fost (1992) puts it: "It is almost beyond comprehension that a typical American consumer, with an 8th-grade reading level, could evaluate such an encyclopedia of information and make an informed choice about whether to undergo prenatal diagnosis and selective abortion, or face an even more complex array of choices regarding gene therapy" (pp. 2815–2816). In sum, mass medical screenings and the universal availability of computers that allow for fast and efficient retrieval, linkage, and processing of medical data threaten to create a society with *medical information overload* that the average citizen may find difficult to cope with in a rational way.

Related to the principle of informed consent is the norm of *telling the truth*. Confidence between health professionals and clients is based on the premise that the information made available to the persons in charge of diagnosis and treatment, e.g., in the form of a test result, should be relayed in a truthful manner to the patient or screenee (Higgs, 1985; Jackson, 1991). Also related is the principle of *autonomy* or lack of paternalism on the part of those providing health care or carrying out research on sick people (Hall, 1992; Westrin, Nilstun, Smedby, & Haglund, 1992). When informing screenees about their test results, their prognosis, the implications of possible elevated risk factors, and what lifestyle changes should be brought about, where exactly does the line go between truth, benevolent deception, and downright lying? Are we justified in portraying risk factors with a certain hype to increase the chances of lifestyle changes and adherence to medical regimens, or is this a form of paternalism and deception that disregards the patient's autonomy and right to make an informed decision about his or her health and future life? As Strecher and Kreuter (Chapter 6) point out, the credibility of health promotion efforts will suffer if one overstates the effects of health behavior changes. Yet these authors themselves argue against using the information obtained at health risk appraisals to arrive at an actual mortality estimate. Instead they argue that the individual's *relative risk* (expressed on an *ordinal* scale) of dying prematurely from a given disease should be focused in the individualized feedback. But what if the absolute risk is infinitesimal even with a greatly increased relative risk? Should not this fact also be conveyed to the user? Indeed, Strecher and Kreuter's second point—that users should be informed about the relative risks of diseases he or she is at risk of acquiring—speaks precisely to the issue of absolute risk (except assuming that these somewhat convoluted absolute risk estimates presumably also are not qualified in the feedback to the user).

When the level of insight and appreciation of the facts of the matter are so unevenly distributed between a screenee and a health professional, there is always the risk that "benevolent" deception and paternalism will get the upper hand. Such a situation is perhaps not very different from what would obtain generally in a doctor-patient relationship, but when large numbers of healthy individuals are enticed to undergo testing and counseling, meticulous respect for the integrity and autonomy of clients is particularly called for. The large-scale nature of screening operations does not necessarily facilitate such observance.

SOME FUTURE PERSPECTIVES

When one moves to "control" behavioral risk factors—for example, quit smoking, drink less alcohol, exercise—the underlying assumption is that the individual is somehow *responsible* for those actions. However, if a medical screening results in the identification of aberrant genes or specific sequences of the DNA known to code for morbidity or premature death a slightly more ambiguous situation arises. Obviously the individual cannot be held responsible for the composition of his or her DNA (although in a not too distant future the parents might). Because of this responsibility-absolving aspect, risk factors rooted in the genetic makeup of the individual may, to a certain extent, be easier to live with.

On the other hand, the experience of having poor luck with respect to one's DNA may lead to fatalism and reduce the potential for positive action. In fact, advances in knowledge about the genetic underpinnings of *health behavior* itself may reintroduce the notion that one is simply a slave of one's genome even at the level of remedial action. If the best research repeatedly shows that there is a very strong genetic component in addictive behaviors such as alcoholism, does not this somehow absolve the drinking person from being personally responsible for his abuse? And would this not be a somewhat unfortunate vantage point if one sets out to modify drinking behavior?

At present there are still several unresolved problems in trying to quantify the proportion of the variance in given behaviors and personality traits (intelligence, extraversion, etc.) that can be attributed to genes. This is particularly true if one sets out to compare across ethnic and racial groups. For example, finding a strong genetic component in intelligence (or addictive behaviors) among both blacks and whites does not necessarily imply that a mean difference between those groups is also genetically rooted. A mean difference may easily be attributed to environmental factors that differ systematically among blacks and whites from birth on (Hedrick, 1985: pp. 551–558). In the wake of the Genome Project and related research, however, our understanding of the link between genotype and phenotype (including morbidity and health behaviors) will move into a new era. Things that previously simply had to be inferred or assumed (e.g., variance at the level of alleles or genes, including epistasis and dominance) in principle will emerge as physical entities that can be correlated with observed illnesses, risk factors, behaviors, and personality traits. In the long run this in turn will provide a far more solid footing for generalizations about the influence of genes and the biological basis of group differences. Thus, at the least, genetic screening operations may contribute to building up a base of knowledge that can have a profound long-term impact on our self-understanding and sense of personal responsibility, both as individuals and as members of ethnic or racial groups (Murray, 1991). Needless to say, the potential for downright racism and stigmatization will grow accordingly.

Such a perspective need not imply that (genetic) screening is undesirable, even if results are used to promote research and knowledge about phenomena that are not directly related to morbidity and mortality. But it points to the necessity of thinking ahead and trying to anticipate the uses and misuses to which information gathered by screening for disease prevention and detection may be put.

REFERENCES

Andrews, L., & Jaeger, A. (1991). Confidentiality of genetic information in the workplace. *American Journal of Law and Medicine, 17*, 75–108.

Aneshensel, C. S., Frerichs, R. R., & Huba, G. J. (1984). Depression and physical illness: a multiwave, nonrecursive causal model. *Journal of Health and Social Behavior, 25*, 350–371.

Barsky, A. J. (1988). The paradox of health. *New England Journal of Medicine, 318*, 414–418.

Beeson, P. B. (1980). Changes in medical therapy during the past half century. *Medicine, 59*, 79–94.

Billings, P. R., Kohn, M. A., de Cuevas, M., Beckwith, J., Alper, J. S., & Natowicz, M. R. (1992). Discrimination as a consequence of genetic screening. *American Journal of Human Genetics, 50*, 476–482.

Childs, B., Gordis, L., Kaback, M. M., & Kazazian, H. G. (1976). Tay Sachs screening: Motives for participating and knowledge of genetics and probability. *American Journal of Human Genetics, 28*, 537–549.

Farrell, P. M., & Mischler, E. H. (1992). Newborn screening for cystic fibrosis. The Cystic Fibrosis Neonatal Screening Study Group. *Advances in Pediatrics, 39*, 35–70.

Fost, N. (1992). Ethical implications of screening asymptomatic individuals. *FASEB Journal, 6*, 2813–2817.

George, L. K., & Landerman, K. (1984). Health and subjective well-being: a replicated secondary data analysis. *International Journal of Aging and Human Development, 19*, 133–156.

Gochfeld, M. (1992). Medical surveillance and screening in the workplace: complementary preventive strategies. *Environmental Research, 59,* 67–80.

Goldberg, D. (1972). *The detection of psychiatric illness by questionnaire.* London: Oxford University Press.

Hall, S. A. (1992). Should public health respect autonomy? *Journal of Medical Ethics, 18,* 197–201.

Hedrick, P. W. (1985). *Genetics of populations.* Boston: Jones and Bartlett Publishers.

Higgs, R. (1985). On telling patients the truth. In M. Lockwood (Ed.), *Moral dilemmas in modern medicine.* Oxford: Oxford University Press.

Hulley, S. B., Newman, T. B., Grady, D., Garber, A. M., Baron, R. B., & Browner, W. S. (1993). Should we be measuring blood cholesterol levels in young adults? *Journal of the American Medical Association, 269,* 1416–1419.

Jackson, J. (1991). Telling the truth. *Journal of Medical Ethics, 17,* 5–9.

Kaplan, G. A., Roberts, R. E., Camacho, T. C., & Coyne, J. C. (1987). Psychosocial predictors of depression. *American Journal of Epidemiology, 125,* 206–220.

Kielstein, R., & Sass, H. M. (1992). Right not to know or duty to know? Prenatal screening for polycystic renal disease. *Journal of Medical Philosophy, 17,* 395–405.

Mann, A. (1984). Hypertension: psychological aspects and diagnostic impact in a clinical trial. *Psychological Medicine Monograph Supplement 5,* 1–35.

Murray, T. H. (1991). Ethical issues in human genome research. *FASEB Journal, 5,* 55–60.

Natowicz, M. R., & Alper, J. S. (1991). Genetic screening: triumphs, problems, and controversies. *Journal of Public Health Policy, 10,* 475–491.

Okun, M. A., Stock, W. A., Haring, M. J., & Witter, R. A. (1984). Health and subjective well-being: A meta-analysis. *International Journal of Aging and Human Development, 19,* 111–132.

Ostrer, H., Allen, W., Crandall, L. A., Moseley, R. E., Dewar, M. A., & Nye, D. (1993). Insurance and genetic testing: Where are we now? *American Journal of Human Genetics, 52,* 565–577.

Rose, G. (1990). British perspective on the U.S. Preventive Services Task Force guidelines. *Journal of General Internal Medicine, 5,* S128–S132.

Terrenoire, G. (1992). Huntington's disease and the ethics of genetic prediction. *Journal of Medical Ethics, 18,* 79–85.

Turner, B. S. (1984). *The body and society.* London: Basil Blackwell.

Tymstra, T. (1991). Prenatal diagnosis, prenatal screening, and the rise of the tentative pregnancy. *International Journal of Technology Assessment and Health Care, 7,* 509–516.

Waltz, J., & Thigpen, C. (1973). Genetic screening and counseling: The legal and ethical issues. *Northwestern University Law Review, 68,* 696–697.

Westrin, C.-G., Nilstun, T., Smedby, B., & Haglund, B. (1992). Epidemiology and moral philosophy. *Journal of Medical Ethics, 18,* 193–196.

Wilfond, B. S., & Fost, N. (1990). The cystic fibrosis gene: Medical and social implications for heterozygote detection. *Journal of the American Medical Association, 263,* 2777–2783.

Index

Abortion, 19, 30
  attitudes toward, 14–15, 18, 194
Absolute risk, 131
Absenteeism, 4, 47–48
Adherence
  in cancer screening, 66–73
  in cholesterol screening, 40, 51–57
AIDS. *See* Human
    immunodeficiency virus
Ambiguity. *See* Uncertainty
Amniocentesis, 15, 17
Anxiety
  about the future, 19
  as a deterrent to screening, 72,
    119
  as a cause of screening, 72
  as a result of screening, 15–17,
    20–21, 47, 66, 70–71, 85–99
  See also Measures; State-Trait
    Anxiety Inventory
Appraisal-behavior relationship,
    172–76
Asbestos, 73–75
Attitudes
  as a result of screening, 18
  toward screening, 12–14, 23, 69
  See also Abortion; Cholesterol, high
Autonomy, 210

Beck Depression Inventory, 24–25
Behavioral Risk Factor Surveillance
    System, 43, 45
Behavioroid measures, 173
Beta-thalassemia. *See*
    Hemoglobinopathies
Breast self-examination, 70–71, 191
Brief Symptom Inventory, 70

Cancer
  genetic susceptibility, 26–27
  impact of screening results, 66–
    69
  See also Adherence; Breast self-
    examination; Mammography;
    Occupational exposures;
    Papanicolaou (Pap) tests
Center for Epidemiological Studies
    Depression Scale, 84–85
Cholesterol, high
  appraisal of, 164–65
  as a risk factor, 39
  attitudes toward control of, 57
  guidelines for, 45–46
  knowledge of, 43–44
  physician practices, 45
  screening technology, 41–42
  strategies for identifying, 39–40
  treatment of, 39
  use of confidence intervals, 42
  See also Dietary change; Memory;
    National Cholesterol Education
    Program; Utilization
Cognitive processing
  in appraisal, 49, 155–58
  of genetic information, 20
Coping styles, 17, 69, 76, 97
  See also Miller Behavioral Style
    Scale
Cystic fibrosis, 14, 17, 21

Deception in research, 146–47
Denial, 25, 42, 49, 74–75, 149–58,
    173–75
  and expectations, 154–55
Depression, 16–17, 24, 84–99

Diagnostic reasoning, 162
Dietary change, 39–40, 44–46, 51–57
    following health risk appraisal,
        134–36
Distress. *See* Anxiety; Depression;
    Fear; Uncertainty
Down syndrome, 16–17, 194

Economic considerations in
    screening, 205–6
Ethnic and cultural factors, 31, 57,
    119–20
Exercise, 98
Experiments, use of, 147–51
    generalizability of, 163–76

False consensus, 161–62
Fatalism, 211
Fear, 3
    of getting AIDS, 97
    fear-drive model, 3
Framing, 76

General Health Questionnaire, 66, 203
General Symptom Index, 24–25
General Well-Being Schedule, 24–25
Genetic counseling, 11, 17, 29
Goal conflict, 28

HD. *See* Huntington's disease
Health Belief Model, 3, 14, 70
    and smoking, 130–32
    applied to health risk appraisal,
        128–33
Health Locus of Control Scale, 67
Health maintenance organizations,
    22, 66
Health risk appraisal
    definition, 126
    prevalence, 126
    recommendations concerning,
        139–41, 190
    validity or estimates, 133
    See also Dietary change; Health
        Belief Model

Hemoglobinopathies, 14, 27, 30
    Beta-thalassemia, 22
    Sickle cell anemia, 4, 20, 31, 204
High blood pressure. *See*
    Hypertension
HIV. *See* Human immunodeficiency
    virus
Hopkins Symptom Checklist, 95
Human immunodeficiency virus
    and the Health Belief Model,
        130–31
    heterosexuals, 119–20
    meaning of test results, 83
    mechanisms of infection, 83
    prevalence of testing for, 83
    See also Measures; Sexual behavior,
        risk-associated
Huntington's disease, 13, 19, 22–26,
    28–31, 185–86
Hypertension, 3, 5, 45, 47, 165–66

Illness stereotypes, 166
Impact of Events Scale, 25, 70
Individual-level effects, 201–4
Informed consent, 21, 209–10
Insurance, 14, 83–84, 203–4, 206–8
    use of data, 48
Interest
    in health behavior change, 131
    in nutrition, 44
    in screening, 13
Intercourse. *See* Sexual behavior
Internal validity, 113

Knowledge
    as a determinant of behavior
        change, 189–90
    as a result of screening, 22, 49–50
    See also Cholesterol, high

Linkage analysis, 23

Mammography, 66–71, 73, 77
Maternal serum alpha fetoprotein, 15,
    17–18, 32

Measures
  of HIV test consequences, 120–21
  psychological, 192–93
  See also Beck Depression Inventory;
    Brief Symptom Inventory;
    Center for Epidemiological
    Studies Depression Scale;
    General Health Questionnaire;
    General Symptom Index;
    General Well-Being Schedule;
    Health Locus of Control Scale;
    Hopkins Symptom Checklist;
    Impact of Events Scale; Miller
    Behavioral Style Scale; Profile of
    Mood States; Social Support
    Questionnaire; State-Trait
    Anxiety Inventory; Zung
    Depression Scale
Medicalization, 208–9
Memory, of cholesterol-related
  information, 49–50
Mental representation, 166
Miller Behavioral Style Scale, 18, 69
Minimization. *See* Denial
Miscarriage, 15
MSAFP. *See* Maternal serum alpha
  fetoprotein

National Cancer Institute, 66
National Cholesterol Education
  Program, 40, 43, 58

Obsessive-compulsive symptoms,
  95
Obstetricians, 14
Occupational exposures, 73–74
Optimism, 21, 72; 134–36

Papanicolaou (Pap) tests, 66, 69, 71,
  73, 77
Partners, 14, 17, 20, 23, 29
  at risk for HIV, 93
  See also Sexual behavior
Personality, 17, 76, 128–29, 171–72,
  211

Persuasion, 3
Profile of Mood States, 18, 67, 85, 94,
  96, 98
Psychological preparation, 25,
  27–28, 188
Psychology, role of in screening
  research, 195–97

Quality-adjusted life years, 201–3

Recessive disorders, 19–22
Regression to the mean, 202–3
Reimbursement for services, 45, 58
Reproductive attitudes and
  decisions, 20–21
  See also Abortion

Scarcity heuristic, 159
Seat belt use, 134–38
Selection bias. *See* Self-selection
Self-efficacy, 130, 132
Self-Regulation Model, 4, 72, 160, 174
Self-selection, 24, 32, 118–19,
  186–87, 202
Sexual behavior
  risk-associated, 99–117
  validity of self-reports, 120–21
Sexual function, 68
Sickle cell anemia. *See*
  Hemoglobinopathies
Sleep patterns, 67–68, 75
Social comparison, 158–60
Social influence, 160–61
Social norms, 117
Social status. *See* Stigmatization
Social support, 17, 24, 118, 138–39
Social Support Questionnaire, 25
Societal-level effects, 205–11
Spouses. *See* Partners
Stages of Change Model. *See*
  Transtheoretical Stages of
  Change Model
State-Trait Anxiety Inventory, 16, 21,
  68, 73, 94, 96
Stigmatization, 20–21, 212

Stress-prevention training, 97
Study designs, 191–92
    See also Experiments, use of
    TAA enzyme paradigm
Suicidal thoughts, 23, 24, 85, 93, 97
Suicide, 23

TAA enzyme paradigm, 147–49
Tay-Sachs disease, 14, 20–21
Theory of Reasoned Action, 4
Transtheoretical Stages of Change
    Model, 3, 141

Uncertainty, 13, 26–28, 31, 47, 68–69,
    168–70, 187
Uptake. *See* Utilization
Utilization, 13–15, 30–31, 43
    of cholesterol screening, 43

Values, 31, 209
Videos, educational, 22, 97

Worksites, 43, 48, 56, 126, 137

Zung Depression Scale, 95